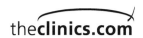

CARDIOLOGY CLINICS

Heart Failure, Part II

GUEST EDITORS
James B. Young, MD
Jagat Narula, MD, PhD

CONSULTING EDITOR
Michael H. Crawford, MD

February 2008 • Volume 26 • Number 1

SAUNDERS

An Imprint of Elsevier, Inc.
PHILADELPHIA   LONDON   TORONTO   MONTREAL   SYDNEY   TOKYO

W.B. SAUNDERS COMPANY
A Division of Elsevier Inc.

Elsevier Inc. • 1600 John F. Kennedy Blvd., Suite 1800 • Philadelphia, Pennsylvania 19103-2899

http://www.theclinics.com

CARDIOLOGY CLINICS
February 2008
Editor: Barbara Cohen-Kligerman

Volume 26, Number 1
ISSN 0733-8651
ISBN-13: 978-1-4160-5780-2
ISBN-10: 1-4160-5780-3

The ideas and opinions expressed in *Cardiology Clinics* do not necessarily reflect those of the Publisher. The Publisher does not assume any responsibility for any injury and/or damage to persons or property arising out of or related to any use of the material contained in this periodical. The reader is advised to check the appropriate medical literature and the product information currently provided by the manufacturer of each drug to be administered to verify the dosage, the method and duration of administration, or contraindications. It is the responsibility of the treating physician or other health care professional, relying on independent experience and knowledge of the patient, to determine drug dosages and the best treatment for the patient. Mention of any product in this issue should not be construed as endorsement by the contributors, editors, or the Publisher of the product or manufacturers' claims.

Cardiology Clinics (ISSN 0733-8651) is published quarterly by Elsevier Inc., 360 Park Avenue South, New York, NY 10010-1710. Months of issue are February, May, August, and November. Business and editorial Offices: 1600 John F. Kennedy Blvd., Suite 1800, Philadelphia, PA 19103 2899. Customer Service Office: 6277 Sea Harbor Drive, Orlando, FL 32887-4800. Periodicals postage paid at New York, NY, and additional mailing offices. Subscription prices are $226.00 per year for US individuals, $344.00 per year for US institutions, $113.00 per year for US students and residents, $276.00 per year for Canadian individuals, $418.00 per year for Canadian institutions, $301.00 per year for international individuals, $418.00 per year for international institutions and $150.00 per year for Canadian and foreign students/residents. To receive student/resident rate, orders must be accompanied by name of affiliated institution, data of term, and the *signature* of program/residency coordinator on institution letterhead. Orders will be billed at individual rate until proof of status is received. Foreign air speed delivery is included in all *Clinics* subscription prices. All prices are subject to change without notice. POSTMASTER: Send address changes to *Cardiology Clinics*, Elsevier Periodicals Customer Service, 6277 Sea Harbor Drive, Orlando, FL 32887-4800. **Customer Service: 1-800-654-2452 (US). From outside of the US, call 1- 407-563-6020. Fax: 1-407-363-9661. E-mail: JournalsCustomerService-usa@elsevier.com.**

Cardiology Clinics is also published in Spanish by McGraw-Hill Interamericana Editores S. A., P.O. Box 5-237, 06500, Mexico D. F., Mexico; in Portuguese by Reichmann and Alfonso Editores Rio de Janeiro, Brazil; and in Greek by Dimitrios P. Lagos, 8 Pondon Street, GR115-28 Ilissia, Greece.

Cardiology Clinics is covered in *Index Medicus, Excerpta Medica, The Cumulative Index to Nursing and Allied Health Literature* (INAHL).

Printed in the United States of America.

CONSULTING EDITOR

MICHAEL H. CRAWFORD, MD, Professor of Medicine, University of California, San Francisco; Lucie Stern Chair in Cardiology, and Interim Chief of Cardiology, University of California San Francisco Medical Center, San Francisco, California; Division of Cardiology, Department of Medicine, University of California, San Francisco Medical Center, San Francisco, California

GUEST EDITORS

JAMES B. YOUNG, MD, Chairman and Professor, Department of Medicine, Lerner College of Medicine; and George and Linda Kaufman Chair, Cleveland Clinic Foundation, Case Western Reserve University, Cleveland, Ohio

JAGAT NARULA, MD, PhD, Professor of Medicine, Chief, Division of Cardiology, University of California, Irvine School of Medicine, Orange, California

CONTRIBUTORS

WILLIAM T. ABRAHAM, MD, FACP, FACC, Professor of Medicine; and Chief, Division of Cardiovascular Medicine, The Ohio State University, Columbus, Ohio

INDER S. ANAND, MD, FRCP, DPhil (OXON), FACC, Professor of Medicine, Division of Cardiology, University of Minnesota Medical School; and Director, Heart Failure Clinic, Veterans Administration Medical Center, Minneapolis, Minnesota

STEFAN D. ANKER, MD, PhD, FESC, Professor, Division of Applied Cachexia Research, Department of Cardiology, Charité Campus Virchow-Klinikum, Berlin, Germany; and Department of Clinical Cardiology, NHLI, Imperial College, London, United Kingdom

JOHN E.A. BLAIR, MD, Fellow, Cardiovascular Diseases, Division of Cardiology, Northwestern University, Feinberg School of Medicine, Chicago, Illinois

FILIPPO BRANDIMARTE, MD, Cardiologist, Department of Cardiovascular, Respiratory and Morphological Sciences, La Sapienza University, Rome, Italy

ANITA DESWAL, MD, MPH, Associate Professor of Medicine, Winters Center for Heart Failure Research, Section of Cardiology, and Houston Center for Quality of Care and Utilization Services, Michael E. DeBakey Veterans Affairs Medical Center and Baylor College of Medicine, Houston, Texas

FRANCESCO FEDELE, MD, Professor of Medicine and Chief, Division of Cardiology and Coronary Care Unit; Director, Fellowship Program, Department of Cardiovascular, Respiratory and Morphological Sciences, La Sapienza University, Rome, Italy

DIMITRIOS FARMAKIS, MD, PhD, Heart Failure Unit and Second Cardiology Department, Attikon University Hospital, Athens, Greece

GERASIMOS FILIPPATOS, MD, PhD, FESC, Assistant Professor, Heart Failure Unit and Second Cardiology Department, Attikon University Hospital, Athens, Greece

VIOREL G. FLOREA, MD, PhD, ScD, FACC, Heart Failure Clinic, Veterans Administration Medical Center; and Cardiology Fellow, Division of Cardiology, University of Minnesota Medical School, Minneapolis, Minnesota

GREGG C. FONAROW, MD, Eliot Corday Professor of Cardiovascular Medicine and Science, Geffen School of Medicine at University of California, Los Angeles (UCLA); and Director, Ahmanson-UCLA Cardiomyopathy Center, UCLA Medical Center, Los Angeles, California

MIHAI GHEORGHIADE, MD, Professor of Medicine and Surgery; Associate Chief, Division of Cardiology; and Director Clinical Service, Department of Internal Medicine, Division of Cardiology, Northwestern University, Feinberg School of Medicine, Chicago, Illinois

SRINIVAS IYENGAR, MD, Clinical Instructor, Division of Cardiology, Columbia University Medical Center, New York, New York

DHRUV KAZI, MD, MSc, Fellow, Section of Cardiology, University of California, San Diego, California

DIMITRIOS T. KREMASTINOS, MD, PhD, FESC, Professor, Heart Failure Unit and Second Cardiology Department, Attikon University Hospital, Athens, Greece

MITJA LAINSCAK, MD, PhD, FESC, The University Clinic of Respiratory and Allergic Diseases Golnik, Heart Failure Unit, Golnik, Slovenia

AMIN MANUCHEHRY, MD, Resident, Internal Medicine, Department of Internal Medicine, Northwestern University, Feinberg School of Medicine, Illinois

DENNIS M. MCNAMARA, MD, Associate Professor of Medicine; and Director, Heart Failure/Transplantation Program, University of Pittsburgh Medical Center, Pittsburgh, Pennsylvania

LESLIE W. MILLER, MD, Washington Hospital Center and Georgetown University, Washington, DC

JOHN T. PARISSIS, MD, PhD, FESC, Heart Failure Unit and Second Cardiology Department, Attikon University Hospital, Athens, Greece

BERTRAM PITT, MD, University of Michigan School of Medicine, Ann Arbor, Michigan

PHILIP A. POOLE-WILSON, MB, MD, FRCP, FMedSci, Professor, Cardiac Medicine, National Heart & Lung Institute, Imperial College London, London, United Kingdom

JONATHAN A. RAPP, MD, Feinberg Cardiovascular Research Institute, Northwestern University Feinberg School of Medicine, Chicago, Illinois

ROBERT L. SCOTT, MD, PhD, FACC, Associate Professor of Medicine; Director, Heart Failure; and Medical Director, Cardiac Transplantation, Mayo Clinic Arizona, Phoenix, Arizona

CONTENTS

III: Management of Chronic Heart Failure (continued from Part I)

> Based on overwhelming data demonstrating reduced morbidity and mortality, ACE inhibitors form a mainstay of therapy in all patients with symptomatic left ventricular systolic dysfunction. Furthermore, ACE inhibitors may be beneficial in the prevention of heart failure in patients with high-risk cardiovascular profiles. However, definite benefit from the use of ACE inhibitors in all patients with heart failure and preserved ejection fraction has not been demonstrated. Even though ACE inhibitors probably have a class effect in patients who have heart failure, it is recommended that ACE inhibitors that have been shown to reduce morbidity and mortality in clinical trials (captopril, enalapril, lisinopril, and ramipril) be used because studies have clearly defined a dose for these agents that is effective in modifying the natural history of the disease. Attempts should be made to up titrate patients to target doses of ACE inhibitors that have been used in clinical trials, if tolerated.

> Aldosterone blockade has been shown to be effective in reducing mortality in patients who have severe heart failure because of systolic left ventricular dysfunction (SLVD) and those who have heart failure and SLVD post–myocardial infarction. Aldosterone blockade also may be beneficial in patients who have New York Heart Association class II heart failure, asymptomatic left ventricular dysfunction, and heart failure with preserved or normal left ventricular function. Considering the beneficial effects of aldosterone blockade on improving nitric oxide availability, endothelial function, and atherosclerosis, it can also be postulated that an aldosterone blockade would add to the benefits of an angiotensin-converting enzyme inhibitor in patients who have coronary artery disease. However, these hypotheses must be confirmed in well-designed, large-scale, prospectively randomized studies.

IV: Management of Post-Myocardial Infarction Left Ventricular Dysfunction

CONTENTS

V: Heart Failure in Perspective

Differences in European and North American Approaches to the Management of Heart Failure
Philip A. Poole-Wilson

In recent years many guidelines on the treatment of specific medical conditions have been published with the goal of advising physicians, promoting good clinical care, and achieving a degree of equity and equality in the delivery of care. Differences exist between European and American guidelines for the management of heart failure not just because of differences in health systems but also because there is little agreement on how to assess clinical trials and convey conclusions in a clear format. Current recommendations can be confusing and often do not reflect the complexities of modern personalized medicine.

Heart Failure: Who We Treat Versus Who We Study
Leslie W. Miller

The prevalence of patients with the diagnosis of heart failure continues to increase, with recent data suggesting that the current estimate in the United States should now be over 7 million patients. There are many sources of information about the patients with heart failure. Many patients have been enrolled in pharmaceutical and devices trials in heart failure, but the patients enrolled are often not reflective of the patients being managed outside of these trials in terms of age, gender, race, and comorbidities. And yet, investigators have extrapolated the results of these trials to all patients with heart failure. This article offers a comparison of the demographics and outcomes of the patients with heart failure that investigators treat and those studied.

Pharmacogenomics for Neurohormonal Intervention in Heart Failure
Dennis M. McNamara

Neurohormonal activation is an important driver of heart failure progression, and all pharmacologic interventions that improve clinical outcomes inhibit this systemic response to myocardial injury. Functional polymorphisms affecting mediator levels and signal transduction are present in genetic loci critical to renin-angiotensin and sympathetic activation. Clinical investigations have demonstrated that these neurohormonal polymorphisms influence heart failure outcomes and alter the effectiveness of drug therapy. Genetic variation of disease modifiers such as angiotensin-converting enzyme (ACE) and β-adrenergic receptors influences ACE inhibitor and β-blocker effectiveness. The investigation of functional genomics will allow pharmacologic therapeutics to be tailored to an individual's specific genetic background. This article explores how genetic variation in genes involved in neurohormonal activation influence heart failure outcomes and the impact of pharmacotherapy.

Index

Part I of Heart Failure was published in the November 2007 issue (Volume 25, Number 4). For the convenience of readers, the table of contents for Part I is shown below.

CONTENTS OF HEART FAILURE, PART I

FORTHCOMING ISSUES

RECENT ISSUES

VISIT OUR WEB SITE

The Clinics are now available online!
Access your subscription at www.theclinics.com

ELSEVIER
SAUNDERS

Cardiol Clin 26 (2008) xi

CARDIOLOGY
CLINICS

Foreword

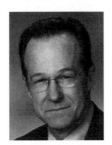

Michael H. Crawford, MD
Consulting Editor

Now that fewer people are dying suddenly of myocardial infarction and ventricular arrhythmias, heart failure is becoming the most frequent cause of cardiac death. Heart failure also has become a major cause of long-term cardiovascular disability. Fortunately, there now are many options to prevent and treat heart failure. Drs. Young and Narula have put together two excellent volumes on this topic. This issue of *Cardiology Clinics* is the second volume on this important topic.

This issue is divided into three sections, each addressing a different area. The first section is a continuation of the discussion begun in volume one about the management of chronic heart failure. The role and optimal dosing of angiotensin-converting enzyme inhibiters are covered. The use of aldosterone inhibition is discussed. The role of neurohormonal therapy in patients who have preserved left ventricular function and heart failure is presented. There is a discussion of neutral endopeptidase inhibitors and endothelin antagonists. Who should receive anticoagulants, antiplatelets, and statin drugs is discussed. Finally, traditional and novel approaches to the management of heart failure are contrasted.

The next section is on management of left ventricular dysfunction after myocardial infarction. One article considers the use of angiotensin-converting enzyme and/or angiotensin receptor blockers after myocardial infarction, and another discusses comprehensive adrenergic blockade for left ventricular dysfunction after myocardial infarction. The last article of this section reviews the role of aldosterone blockade in patients who have left ventricular dysfunction after acute myocardial infarction.

The final section includes a discussion of the difference between the European and American approaches to heart failure and what these differences mean for the care of our patients. Heart failure trials are put into perspective, because patients seen in clinical practice are not always similar to those enrolled in trials. The issue ends with a look to the future of pharmacogenetics for neurohormonal interventions in heart failure.

The international authors who contributed to this issue provide considerable insights into these complex issues. I learned a lot from them, and I know you will as well.

Michael H. Crawford, MD
Division of Cardiology, Department of Medicine
University of California
San Francisco Medical Center
505 Parnassus Avenue, Box 0124
San Francisco, CA 94143-0124, USA

E-mail address: crawfordm@medicine.ucsf.edu

doi:10.1016/j.ccl.2008.01.002

cardiology.theclinics.com

ELSEVIER
SAUNDERS

Cardiol Clin 26 (2008) 1–14

CARDIOLOGY
CLINICS

Role and Optimal Dosing of Angiotensin-Converting Enzyme Inhibitors in Heart Failure

Dhruv Kazi, MD, MSc[a], Anita Deswal, MD, MPH[b],*

[a]Division of Cardiology, University of California, 200 W Arbor Drive, MPF 360, San Diego, CA 92103, USA
[b]Winters Center for Heart Failure Research, Section of Cardiology, and Houston Center of Quality of Care
and Utilization Services, Michael E. DeBakey Veterans Affairs Medical Center (111B) and Baylor College
of Medicine, 2002 Holcombe Boulevard, Houston, TX 77030, USA

An understanding of the important role of neurohormonal up-regulation in disease progression in heart failure has been translated into therapeutic strategies using neurohormonal antagonists to improve cardiac function, alter disease progression, and improve survival. Angiotensin-converting enzyme (ACE) inhibitors, which were the first of this class of drugs proved to alter the natural history of heart failure and lead to long-term benefit, remain a cornerstone of therapy in all stages of heart failure. This article reviews the rationale for their use, key clinical trial data supporting the major role of ACE inhibitors in heart failure, and the recommended dosing in this patient population.

Rationale for the use of angiotensin-converting enzyme inhibitors in heart failure

Activation of the renin-angiotensin system plays a critical role in the pathogenesis of heart failure [1]. The deleterious effects of renin-angiotensin system activation in heart failure are mediated primarily through increased circulating and tissue levels of the neurohormone angiotensin II. Angiotensin II is an extremely potent vasoconstrictor, acting directly on vascular smooth muscles and indirectly by increasing sympathetic

tone [2,3]. In addition, it produces sodium retention (through aldosterone and renal vasoconstriction), as well as fluid retention (through antidiuretic hormone) [4,5]. At the cellular level, angiotensin II promotes migration, proliferation, and hypertrophy, thus producing numerous adverse effects, including remodeling of the left ventricle, alterations in the morphology and mechanical properties of the vasculature, and the development of endothelial dysfunction [6,7].

Angiotensin II promotes cardiac remodeling in several ways. By increasing arterial smooth muscle tone and causing salt and water retention, it increases cardiac preload and afterload, and increased wall stress is a potent stimulus for remodeling. In addition, angiotensin II has direct effects on the myocardium, causes hypertrophy of cardiac myocytes and hyperplasia of cardiac fibroblasts associated with an increase in extracellular matrix deposition [8], and stimulates the release of other growth factors, including norepinephrine and endothelin, which in turn stimulate cardiac remodeling [9]. These actions of angiotensin II are mediated largely through the angiotensin type 1 (AT1) receptor.

The renin-angiotensin system may be inhibited at various levels, as shown in Fig. 1. ACE inhibitors block the action of ACE, the enzyme responsible for the conversion of angiotensin I to angiotensin II, thereby reducing the angiotensin II available to stimulate the angiotensin receptors. Thus, ACE inhibition attenuates many of the key hemodynamic, mechanical, and functional disturbances crucial to the pathophysiology of heart failure. In addition to its ACE blocking effects,

This article is supported in part by grants from the VA Health Services Research and Development Service (IIR 02-082-1) and the VA Clinical Science Research and Development Service.

A version of this article originally appeared in Heart Failure Clinics, volume 1, issue 1.

* Corresponding author.

E-mail address: adeswal@bcm.tmc.edu (A. Deswal).

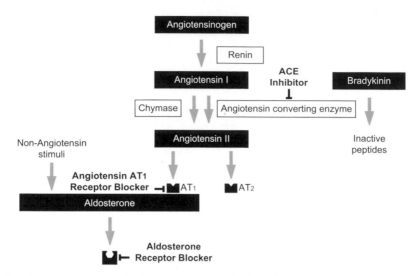

Fig. 1. Activation of the renin-angiotensin-aldosterone system. Angiotensin (AT) is converted to angiotensin I (ATI) by renin. ATI can be converted to angiotensin II (ATII) through ACE and chymase-dependent pathways. ATII exerts its biological effects by binding to AT receptors. Aldosterone production is stimulated by ATII as well as by AT-independent mechanisms. ACE inhibitors block ACE-dependent conversion of ATI to ATII. ACE inhibitors also prevent the catabolism of bradykinin, which can lead to an increase in the local generation of nitric oxide and prostaglandins.

ACE also catalyzes the degradation of bradykinin (see Fig. 1). Bradykinin has direct and indirect vasodilator activity mediated by release of nitric oxide and prostaglandin, as well as antimitotic and antithrombotic actions that could be of benefit in heart failure [10]. It also causes natriuresis by a direct tubular effect in the kidney [11]. ACE inhibition results in an accumulation of kinins and accentuation of kinin-mediated prostaglandin synthesis, and experimental data have shown that the hemodynamic and remodeling modification response to ACE inhibition is attenuated significantly by the simultaneous administration of a bradykinin antagonist [12,13]. Thus, in addition to blocking the production of angiotensin II, the therapeutic effects of ACE inhibition in patients who have heart failure may be caused in part by its effect on the kallikrein-kinin system and the attendant increase in endogenous kinin levels.

Although first developed as antihypertensive agents, ACE inhibitors occupy a central role in the management of heart failure [7,14]. Initially, the hemodynamic effects of ACE inhibitors were believed to be central to their role in heart failure. They were expected to optimize loading conditions imposed on the failing heart by reducing peripheral vascular resistance, thus enhancing cardiac output. Studies with the ACE inhibitor captopril demonstrated an increase in cardiac output, lowering of left ventricular (LV) filling pressures, and modest reductions in systolic blood pressure and heart rate in patients who had heart failure and LV systolic dysfunction. These effects were sustained with long-term ACE inhibition [15–17]. It has since been recognized that the effect of ACE inhibitors on LV remodeling may be one of the most important mechanisms for their efficacy in patients who have heart failure [18]. Recently, it has been recognized increasingly that the antiatherogenic, anti-inflammatory, antiproliferative, and antithrombotic properties of ACE inhibitors likely contribute to the vascular protective effects noted in patients with and without heart failure [19,20].

Angiotensin-converting enzyme inhibitors in symptomatic heart failure: evidence from clinical trials

A large body of evidence supports the use of ACE inhibitors in heart failure: ACE inhibitors have been evaluated in clinical trials of more than 7000 patients who have symptomatic heart failure. A meta-analysis based on 7105 patients from 32 published and unpublished trials investigated the efficacy of ACE inhibition in patients who have heart failure [21]. All patients in the analysis had symptomatic heart failure (New York Heart Association [NYHA] functional class II–IV), LV systolic dysfunction, or limitation of exercise duration. In most trials, patients were on background therapy with either digoxin and diuretics or only diuretics. Of these 32 trials, 28 trials with 6726 patients used captopril, enalapril, ramipril, quinapril, or lisinopril. The remaining agents, benazepril hydrochloride, cilazapril, and perindopril, were used in 379 patients. ACE inhibitors significantly reduced mortality (odds ratio [OR] 0.77; 95% confidence interval [CI] 0.67–0.88), which was caused chiefly by a substantial reduction in deaths attributable to progressive heart failure (OR 0.69; 95% CI 0.58–0.83; $P < .001$); point estimates for effects on sudden or presumed arrhythmic deaths and fatal myocardial infarction were not significant. The odds of developing the combined endpoint of death or hospitalization for heart failure were 0.65 (95% CI 0.57–0.74), and there was no evidence of heterogeneity across the different agents. In addition, there were significant reductions in myocardial infarction and nonsignificant reductions in strokes and other thromboembolic events.

Although most of the effect was noted in the first 90 days of treatment, additional benefit continued to accrue with longer use. Most trials were short with duration of 3 months; 12 trials had patient follow-up beyond 90 days. The reductions in total mortality and the combined endpoint of total mortality or hospitalization for

heart failure were consistent in the various subgroups based on age, sex, NYHA class, and etiology, although the patients with greater LV systolic dysfunction (LV ejection fraction [LVEF] ≤ 25%) benefited the most. The largest amount of data was from the trials using enalapril, in which there was a significant reduction in mortality (Table 1). Although the reductions in mortality were not statistically significant in the trials using captopril, ramipril, quinapril, and lisinopril, the point estimates were consistent with the overall effect of enalapril (see Table 1). Thus these trials have established the role of ACE inhibitors in reducing mortality and heart failure hospitalization in patients who have heart failure.

Salient features of the three landmark trials with ACE inhibitors in symptomatic heart failure— the Studies of Left Ventricular Dysfunction (SOLVD) treatment trial, the Cooperative North Scandinavian Enalapril Survival Study (CONSENSUS), and the Veterans Administration Cooperative Vasodilator-Heart Failure Trial II (V-HeFT II)—are detailed in Table 2. These trials were included in the meta-analysis discussed above and individually established the role of the ACE inhibitor enalapril in prolonging survival in patients with the complete range of symptomatic heart failure (NYHA class II–IV) secondary to LV systolic dysfunction [22–24].

Table 1
Total mortality or hospitalization for heart failure by duration of follow-up and agent for randomized trials of angiotensin-converting enzyme inhibitors

Agent	No. of trials	ACE inhibitors (no. of events/no. randomized)	Controls(no. of events/no. randomized)	OR (95% CI)
90 days or less of follow-up				
Captopril	4	27/292	42/288	0.60 (0.36–1.00)
Enalapril	7	157/1690	259/1691	0.52 (0.42–0.65)
Lisinopril	4	10/351	10/195	0.50 (0.19–1.27)
Quinapril	5	3/548	3/327	0.68 (0.13–3.66)
Ramipril	6	33/714	44/513	0.52 (0.32–0.83)
All other trials	4	9/215	14/164	0.51 (0.21–1.24)
Total	30	239/3810	372/3178	0.53 (0.44–0.63)
More than 90 days of follow-up				
Captopril	3	52/214	66/206	0.68 (0.44–1.04)
Enalapril	3	559/1282	592/1187	0.78 (0.66–0.91)
Lisinopril	0	—	—	—
Quinapril	2	2/218	2/210	0.96 (0.14–6.87)
Ramipril	2	2/120	3/83	0.58 (0.10–3.48)
Total	10	615/1834	663/1686	0.76 (0.66–0.88)

Data from Garg R, Yusuf S. Overview of randomized trials of angiotensin-converting enzyme inhibitors on mortality and morbidity in patients with heart failure. Collaborative Group on ACE Inhibitor Trials. JAMA 1995;273(18):1450–6.

Table 2
Selected clinical trials establishing the benefit of angiotensin-converting enzyme inhibitors in symptomatic and asymptomatic left ventricular systolic dysfunction

Trial [Ref.] (no. of patients; average follow-up)	Study population	ACE inhibitor and dose	Key results
CONSENSUS I [22] (n = 253; 6 mo)	NYHA IV	Enalapril versus placebo 2.5 mgtwice daily titrated to 20 mg twice daily	6-mo mortality decreased 40% 1-y mortality decreased 31% Improvement in NYHA class Decrease in cardiac size
V-HeFT II [24] (n = 804; 2.5 y)	NYHA II– IV LVEF <45%	Target enalapril 10 mg twice daily versus hydralazine 75 mg four times daily + isosorbide dinitrate 40 mg four times daily	2-y mortality decreased 28% No difference in HF hospitalization Lesser improvement in exercise capacity and ventricular function with enalapril
SOLVD Treatment Trial [23] (n = 2569; 41 mo)	NYHA II–IV (90% II–III) LVEF ≤ 35%	Enalapril versus placebo 2.5 mg twice daily titrated to 10 mg twice daily	16% decrease in mortality 22% decrease in progressive HF mortality 26% decrease in either death or HF hospitalization 8.6-mo increase in median life expectancy [77]
SOLVD Prevention Trial [30] (n = 4228; 37.4 mo)	NYHA I LVEF ≤ 35%	Enalapril versus placebo 2.5 mg twice daily titrated to 10 mg twice daily	20% decrease in either death or HF hospitalization 29% decrease in either death or development of HF

In addition to their benefit on mortality, several trials have shown that ACE inhibitors improve symptoms and exercise capacity in patients who have heart failure. Narang and colleagues [25] reviewed 35 published, double-blind, randomized placebo-controlled trials involving 3411 patients that compared the effect of ACE inhibitors and placebo on exercise capacity in patients who had symptomatic chronic heart failure. Exercise duration improved in 23 of the studies, whereas symptoms improved in 25 of the 33 studies that evaluated this. In most trials (27 of 33), there was concordance between the effect on symptoms and on exercise capacity, but six trials showed discrepant results. All nine trials with sample size more than 50, follow-up of 3 to 6 months, and use of treadmill exercise tests showed improved exercise capacity as well as symptoms.

Data on the use of ACE-inhibition in patients with symptomatic heart failure and preserved ejection fraction are limited. The Perindopril in Elderly People with Chronic Heart Failure (PEP-CHF) study was a randomized, double-blind, placebo controlled trial evaluating the use of the ACE inhibitor, perindopril, in elderly patients with symptomatic heart failure, preserved LVEF

and evidence of diastolic dysfunction [26]. The power of the study was substantially reduced by slow enrollment, lower than expected event rates, and substantial attrition during the course of the study. At the end of the study, there was no significant difference between the perindopril and placebo groups in mortality or heart failure hospitalization, the composite primary endpoint of the study (hazard ratio 0.92, 95% CI 0.70-1.21). However, a large number of patients stopped their assigned treatment after the first year and started taking open label ACE inhibitors. If analysis was confined to the first year, perindopril was associated with a lower event rate, with a reduction in the primary end point (hazard ratio 0.69, 95% CI 0.47, 1.01, P = .055), a reduction in heart failure hospitalization (hazard ratio 0.63, 95% CI 0.41, 0.97, P = .033), improved NYHA class (P<.03) and an improvement in 6 minute walk distance. In summary, the trial did not show a statistical benefit of ACE inhibitors on long-term morbidity or mortality in patients with heart failure and preserved ejection fraction, but did suggest some improvement in symptoms and exercise capacity and possibly heart failure hospitalizations in this patient population.

Angiotensin-converting enzyme inhibitors in asymptomatic left ventricular systolic dysfunction

Patients who have asymptomatic LV dysfunction are at high risk for developing heart failure and for death [27]. Studies have shown some degree of neurohormonal activation in patients who have asymptomatic LV dysfunction and mild heart failure, and that this activation may be more marked during exercise [28,29]. These factors led to the evaluation of the effect of ACE inhibitors on morbidity, mortality, and development of heart failure in patients who have asymptomatic LV systolic dysfunction in the SOLVD Prevention Trial [30]. In this trial of asymptomatic patients with depressed LVEF who were not receiving any therapy for heart failure, enalapril significantly reduced the rate of the combined endpoint of death or hospitalization for heart failure and significantly delayed the development of heart failure (see Table 2). Enalapril produced an 8%, nonsignificant reduction in mortality ($P = .30$), however. Notably, 41% of all patients in the placebo group and 51% of patients in the placebo group who were hospitalized for heart failure were prescribed an open-label ACE inhibitor, suggesting an underestimation of the effect of ACE inhibition in patients who have asymptomatic LV systolic dysfunction. Thus, in a patient population with asymptomatic LV dysfunction, ACE inhibitors were associated with a significant benefit on morbidity but not on mortality. A substudy demonstrated that chronic ACE inhibition resulted in slowing or reversal of LV dilatation in patients who had asymptomatic LV dysfunction, suggesting that as in systolic heart failure, the clinical benefits of ACE inhibition may have been caused in part by its impact on ventricular remodeling [31].

Angiotensin-converting enzyme inhibition in patients who have heart failure or left ventricular systolic dysfunction post–myocardial infarction

There is a marked increase in fatal and nonfatal cardiovascular events among survivors of acute myocardial infarction [32], with the degree of LV dysfunction being the most important determinant of the increased risk [33,34]. After the initial insult, residual viable myocardium undergoes progressive remodeling and dilatation, leading to deterioration in LV performance [35–37]. The degree of LV dysfunction is proportionate to the size and age of the scar. Animal experiments as well as clinical studies with surrogate endpoints (ventricular size and function) have demonstrated the efficacy of ACE inhibition in the attenuation of LV dilatation and progressive LV dysfunction [18,38,39]. In addition, ACE inhibitors may have antiatherogenic, anti-inflammatory, antiproliferative, and antithrombotic effects that may reduce recurrent myocardial infarction in these patients [19,20].

The three long-term trials that demonstrated benefit of the ACE inhibitors captopril, ramipril, and trandolapril in patients who had LV systolic dysfunction or heart failure after an acute myocardial infarction are detailed in Table 3 [32,40,41]. An overview of these three trials established that the use of ACE-inhibitor therapy, begun within 3 to 16 days after an acute myocardial infarction and continued long-term, was associated with an overall reduction in mortality (OR 0.74; 95% CI 0.66–0.83), recurrent myocardial infarction (OR 0.80; 95% CI 0.69–0.94), hospitalization for heart failure (OR 0.73; 95% CI 0.63–0.85), and development of heart failure [42]. The results indicated that 15 patients would need to be treated for 2.5 years to prevent one death. Long-term follow-up of patients in two of these trials also demonstrated a sustained benefit on survival [43,44].

Angiotensin-converting enzyme inhibition and prevention of heart failure in patients without left ventricular systolic dysfunction

Having demonstrated the efficacy of ACE inhibitors in patients who have LV systolic dysfunction, irrespective of clinical symptoms of heart failure, the next logical step was to investigate their role in the prevention of heart failure in patients without LV systolic dysfunction, in patients who have hypertension, for example, or in patients at high risk for cardiovascular events. In patients who have hypertension, ACE inhibitors may prevent or delay the progression of myocardial fibrosis and structural disarray in the hypertensive heart by blunting the renin-angiotensin system over a prolonged period, and thus may prevent or delay the onset of heart failure [45,46].

A recent meta-analysis of six trials of antihypertensive therapy evaluated the benefits of ACE inhibitors versus all other antihypertensive agents (including diuretics, beta blockers, calcium

Table 3
Selected clinical trials establishing the benefit of angiotensin-converting enzyme inhibitors after an acute myocardial
infarction

Trial [Ref.] (no. of patients; average follow-up)	Study population	ACE inhibitor and dose	Key results
SAVE [32] (n = 2231; 42 mo)	3–16 d post-MI LVEF<40% No overt HF	Captopril 12.5 mg three times daily titrated to 50 mg three times daily	19% decrease in all-cause mortality 21% decrease in CV mortality 37% decrease in severe HF 25% decrease in recurrent MI
AIRE [41,44] (n = 2006; 15 mo)	3–10 d post-MI Clinical HF irrespective of LVEF	Ramipril 2.5 mg twice daily titrated 5 mg twice daily	27% decrease in all cause mortality 19% decrease in death, reinfarction, severe HF, or stroke 23% decrease in severe HF 30% decrease in sudden death No effect on recurrent MI
TRACE [40] (n = 2606; 36 mo)	3–7 d post-MI Wall motion index ≤ 1.2 LVEF ≤ 35%	Trandolapril 1 mg once daily titrated up to 4 mg once daily	22% decrease in all-cause mortality 25% decrease in CV mortality 29% decrease in severe HF 24% decrease in sudden death

Abbreviations: CV, cardiovascular; HF, heart failure; MI, myocardial infarction.

channel blockers, and alpha blockers) [47]. The main finding of this analysis was that the risk for heart failure did not differ between patients randomized to receive ACE inhibitors and those randomized to receive other classes of antihypertensives (Fig. 2). This analysis assumed, however, that all other antihypertensive agents evaluated were equal in their effects on the development of heart failure. Using the same trials, but evaluating ACE inhibitors against individual drug classes (diuretics, beta blockers, calcium channel blockers, and beta blocker and diuretic combination) yielded slightly different results [48]. As shown in Fig. 2, although diuretics seemed superior to or no different than ACE inhibitors (OR for ACE inhibitors versus other drugs 1.07; 95% CI 0.80–1.43) in the prevention of heart failure, ACE inhibitors seemed superior to calcium channel blockers in preventing heart failure (OR 0.84; 95% CI 0.76–0.93). Based on these data, one may conclude that in a general population with hypertension, ACE inhibitors may not have a consistent benefit in preventing heart failure, but may be superior to calcium channel blockers.

Results were different, however, in patients who were at high risk for the development of cardiovascular events. The Heart Outcome Evaluation Project (HOPE) examined benefit of the ACE inhibitor ramipril in reducing mortality and morbidity in high-risk patients without heart failure or known depressed LVEF [49]. A total of 9297 elderly patients (> 55 years of age) with a history of coronary artery disease, stroke, peripheral vascular disease, or diabetes mellitus plus at least one other cardiovascular risk factor (hypertension, elevated total cholesterol levels, low high-density lipoprotein cholesterol levels, cigarette smoking, or documented microalbuminuria) were randomized to receive either ramipril at a target dose of 10 mg/d or placebo for an average of 5 years. Overall, patients in the ramipril group had a 22% reduction in the primary composite outcome of myocardial infarctions, stroke, or death from cardiovascular causes. In addition, the allocation to treatment with ramipril significantly reduced the rate of all heart failure (composite of heart failure death, heart failure requiring hospitalization, heart failure requiring ACE inhibitor, or any reported heart failure) by 23% and the rate of combined cardiovascular death and all heart failure by 24% [50]. When analyzed separately, each component of the composite endpoint of heart failure showed benefit with ramipril. Documentation of LVEF was not required for entry into the study, but of 5193

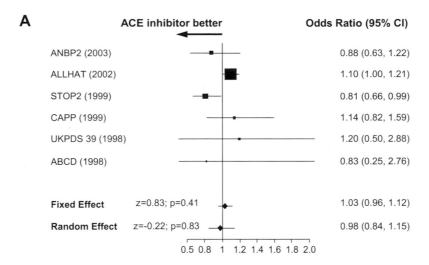

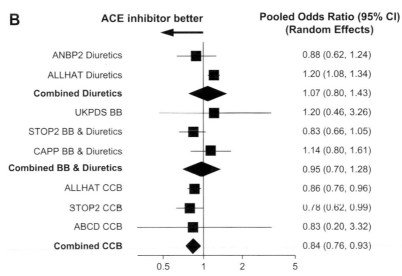

Fig. 2. (A) Meta-analysis of effectiveness of ACE inhibitors in the prevention of heart failure in patients who have hypertension: comparison of ACE inhibitors to all other drugs. ABCD, Appropriate Blood Pressure Control in Diabetes; ANBP2, Second Australian National Blood Pressure Project; ALLHAT, Antihypertensive and Lipid-Lowering Treatment to Prevent Heart Attack Trial; CAPP, Captopril Prevention Project; STOP-2, Swedish Trial in Old Patients with Hypertension-2; UKPDS, UK Prospective Diabetes Study Group. (*From* Angeli F, Verdecchia P, Reboldi GP, et al. Meta-analysis of effectiveness or lack thereof of angiotensin-converting enzyme inhibitors for prevention of heart failure in patients with systemic hypertension. Am J Cardiol 2004;93(2):240 3; with permission.) (*B*) Meta-analysis of effectiveness of ACE inhibitors in the prevention of heart failure in patients who have hypertension: comparison of ACE inhibitors to other drug classes. (*From* Mills E, Montori VM, Thabane L. Angiotensin-converting enzyme inhibitor meta-analysis provides misleading conclusion. Am J Cardiol 2004; 94(1):149; with permission.)

patients who had known LVEF at baseline, 92% had a normal LVEF and a subgroup analysis of patients who had documented normal LVEF at baseline (n = 4775) found similar benefits to those seen in the overall group. The benefits of ramipril on heart failure development were consistent across most subgroups. There was a significant interaction between baseline blood pressure and treatment group. Ramipril was associated with a 9% reduction in heart failure in patients who had baseline systolic blood pressure below the median (139 mm Hg) compared with a larger 33%

reduction in patients who had blood pressure above the median. Thus, mechanisms for prevention of heart failure in patients at high risk could include better control of blood pressure in addition to prevention of myocardial infarction, as well as beneficial effects in diabetics with ACE inhibition [50]. The benefit of ACE inhibitors in reducing hospitalizations for heart failure in a population with atherosclerosis but without heart failure or reduced LVEF at baseline has also since been confirmed in a meta-analysis of three large trials including the HOPE trial [51].

Choice of angiotensin-converting enzyme inhibitors and optimal dosing

Although most evidence supporting an effect of ACE inhibitors on the survival of patients who have symptomatic heart failure is derived from experience with enalapril, the available data suggest that there are no differences among available ACE inhibitors in their effects on symptoms or survival (see Table 1) [21]. It has been suggested that drugs in this class may differ in their ability to inhibit tissue ACE, but no trial has shown that tissue ACE-inhibiting agents are superior to other ACE inhibitors in any clinical aspect of heart failure. In selecting among ACE inhibitors, however, it is recommended that preference be given to ACE inhibitors that reduced morbidity and mortality in clinical trials (eg, captopril, enalapril, lisinopril, and ramipril), because such studies have defined a dose that effectively modifies the natural history of the disease. Such information generally is lacking for ACE inhibitors that were not evaluated in large-scale studies [52].

Despite overwhelming evidence of the benefits of ACE inhibitors on morbidity and mortality in heart failure, initial surveys reflected significant underuse as well as use of doses much lower than those used in clinical trials. This may be based on the perception that the degree of benefit accrued depends on the use of ACE inhibitors (irrespective of their dose), whereas the adverse events are dose-dependent, although these assumptions have not been validated [53]. Additionally, there is a marked reluctance to initiate or advance therapy in patients who have baseline hypotension or renal insufficiency or in elderly patients, despite evidence that these patients receive as much benefit from the ACE inhibitor therapy as other patients [54–56]. Because many patients are treated at doses below the target

doses used in clinical trials, there remains significant interest in whether lower doses of ACE inhibitors confer similar reductions in morbidity and mortality.

Earlier clinical studies showed that higher doses of ACE inhibitors offered greater hemodynamic [16,57,58] and symptomatic [59] benefit compared with lower doses, and experimental data indicated reduction in mortality with higher doses of ACE inhibition in animal models [60]. Therefore, clinical studies were performed to evaluate the use of ACE inhibitors at low dose, at target doses used in large clinical trials, and at higher than target doses.

Tang and colleagues [61] compared the neurohormonal responses and clinical effects of high-dose (40 mg/d) versus low-dose (5 mg/d) enalapril over 6 months in 75 patients who had chronic heart failure and LV systolic dysfunction. In the 48 patients who remained in the study at the end of 6 months, high-dose enalapril was associated with a greater reduction in serum ACE activity compared with the low-dose group. High-dose enalapril was not associated with greater suppression of angiotensin II, aldosterone, or norepinephrine levels, however. There were nearly twice the number of predetermined clinical events including emergency room visits, hospital admissions, deaths, and sustained increases in diuretic doses in the low-dose group compared with the high-dose group (53% versus 30%), but this finding did not reach statistical significance ($P = .06$). Similarly, a trend toward a greater reduction in LV diastolic dimensions was noted in the high-dose arm ($P = .08$). Enalapril was well tolerated even at the high doses. More adverse events were reported in the low-dose group than in the high-dose group.

Conversely, the NETWORK study of 1532 patients, which compared low-dose (2.5 mg twice daily), intermediate (5 mg twice daily), or high-dose (10 mg twice daily) enalapril for 6 months, found no significant differences in mortality or hospitalization among the three groups. It should be noted, however, that this study was of short duration and overall only had 53 deaths and 90 hospitalizations for heart failure in the randomized patients, thus allowing suboptimal power for detection of smaller differences between groups [62]. Nanas and colleagues [63] took a different approach. They compared differences in survival, clinical, and hemodynamic variables between patients treated with either standard dose (target 20 mg/d; mean dose achieved 17.9 ± 4.3

mg/d) or higher than standard dose (target 60 mg/d; mean dose achieved 42 ± 19.3 mg/d) enalapril in 248 patients. At the end of 1 year of follow-up, they found no significant differences in survival or in clinical or hemodynamic variables between the two groups. Thus, these smaller studies did not define clearly the importance of ACE-inhibitor dosing in patients who have heart failure on mortality, morbidity, or exercise tolerance [64].

The Assessment of Treatment with Lisinopril and Survival (ATLAS) Trial was performed with the objective of definitively comparing the efficacy and safety of low- versus high-dose ACE inhibition on mortality and morbidity in chronic heart failure [65]. The ATLAS trial randomized 3164 patients with LVEF ≤ 30% and chronic heart failure (NYHA II–IV) to either low-dose (target 2.5–5.0 mg/d) or high-dose (target 32.5–35.0 mg/d) of the ACE inhibitor lisinopril. This dose selection was based on previous studies that showed the lower dose of 2.5 to 5 mg of lisinopril to have favorable hemodynamic effects [58], whereas doses of lisinopril, 20 to 40 mg/d, were comparable to the doses of ACE inhibitors that had demonstrated beneficial effects on morbidity and mortality in prior clinical trials [65,66]. The trial had an initial open-label phase for at least 4 weeks in which an attempt was made to up-titrate to and maintain patients at lisinopril, 12.5 mg/d to 15 mg/d. Almost 5% of patients were excluded from participation in the trial because they could not tolerate the intermediate doses of lisinopril during this open-label period. Of the 3164 patients that were randomized, 93% achieved target dose in the low-dose group and 91% achieved target dose in the high-dose group. During the course of the study, 31% of patients in the low dose and 27% patients in the high-dose group discontinued therapy. In addition, 22% of patients in the low-dose and 18% of the high-dose group were started on open label therapy, potentially decreasing the magnitude of differences in benefit between the two groups.

After a median follow-up of 46 months, compared with the low-dose group, patients receiving the higher dose of lisinopril had a non-significant 8% reduction in all-cause mortality ($P = .128$), a 10% reduction in cardiovascular mortality ($P = .073$) and a 12% reduction in the combined endpoint of all-cause mortality or hospitalization for any reason ($P = .002$). Patients on high-dose lisinopril, however, had 24% fewer hospitalizations for heart failure ($P = .002$), 13% reduction in all-cause hospitalizations ($P = .021$),

and 16% reduction in cardiovascular hospitalizations ($P = .05$). This study also demonstrated the relative safety of high-dose ACE inhibition. Although high-dose lisinopril was associated with more frequent dizziness, hypotension, mild decrease in renal function, and hyperkalemia, these side effects did not lead patients to stop the study medication more frequently in the high-dose group than in the low-dose group (17% versus 18%). Compared with the low-dose group, fewer patients in the high-dose group experienced cough or reported worsening heart failure as an adverse event [65].

Thus the ATLAS trial demonstrated that when compared with low doses of ACE inhibitors, the use of high doses reduces the risk for major clinical events, especially cardiovascular and heart failure hospitalizations. This can translate into significant cost savings as well as improvement in quality of life. There was no significant reduction in all-cause mortality with the use of high-dose ACE inhibitors, however. The benefit achieved with low-dose ACE inhibition compared with high-dose inhibition was approximately half that noted when comparable high-dose ACE inhibitors were compared with placebo in the SOLVD studies [23], suggesting that low-dose ACE inhibitors may provide about half the benefits associated with the high dose of these agents. Also, the study results do not clarify whether there is any incremental benefit from intermediate to high-dose ACE inhibition [65].

Therefore, available data support trying to up-titrate ACE inhibitor doses beyond the low doses, if tolerated. Until further data are available, it may be prudent to attempt up-titration to the target doses shown beneficial in clinical trials of ACE inhibitors in patients who have heart failure [52]. If target doses of an ACE inhibitor cannot be tolerated, lower doses should be used with the expectation that the lower doses exert benefit, albeit less than higher doses. Table 4 lists the initial and target doses of ACE inhibitors that are recommended in the treatment of patients who have heart failure.

Patient characteristics as a determinant of benefit from angiotensin-converting enzyme inhibition

Although the numerous clinical trials of ACE inhibition in patients who have heart failure provide incontrovertible evidence in its favor, it is unclear whether this benefit extends equally

Table 4
Recommended doses of angiotensin-converting enzyme inhibitors in heart failure

Drug	Initial dose	Target/maximum dose
Captopril	6.25 mg three times daily	50 mg three times daily
Enalapril	2.5 mg twice daily	10 to 20 mg twice daily
Fosinopril	5 to 10 mg once daily	40 mg once daily
Lisinopril	2.5 to 5.0 mg once daily	20 to 40 mg once daily
Quinapril	10 mg twice daily	40 mg twice daily
Ramipril	1.25 to 2.5 mg once daily	10 mg once daily
Perindopril	2 mg once daily	8 to 16 mg once daily
Trandolapril	1 mg once daily	4 mg once daily

Data from Hunt SA, Abraham WT, Chin MH et al. ACC/AHA Guideline Update for the Diagnosis and Management of Chronic Heart Failure in the Adult. J Am Coll Cardiol. 2005 Sep 20;46(6):e1–82.

across all subgroups. This section discusses various patient characteristics that may influence the degree of benefit achieved from ACE inhibitors.

Disease severity

In most clinical trials of ACE inhibition in heart failure, patients who had greater severity of clinical heart failure and lower LVEF obtained the greatest benefit. The CONSENSUS trial demonstrated a 31% reduction in mortality in patients who had NYHA class-IV heart failure after treatment with enalapril for 6 months, whereas the SOLVD treatment trial, which predominantly included patients in NYHA class II and III, demonstrated a 16% reduction in mortality at 41 months [22,23]. On a similar note, the SOLVD prevention trial, which looked at patients with asymptomatic LV dysfunction, produced only an 8% nonsignificant trend toward reduced mortality with enalapril [30].

Patients who have hyponatremia (serum sodium < 135 mEq/L) tend to be more sensitive to ACE inhibition, likely because of higher plasma renin levels [67]. Hyponatremia identifies patients more likely to develop hypotension and worsening azotemia after the initiation of ACE inhibitors.

Baseline azotemia identifies a group of patients at increased risk for all-cause mortality in patients who have heart failure [68,69]. On the other hand,

some patients are at a higher risk for deterioration of renal function after initiation of an ACE inhibitor, particularly those who are older or on diuretics [70]. It is therefore imperative to start at a low dose and up-titrate the dose cautiously in patients who have pre-existing renal disease with close monitoring of renal function and serum potassium during the initiation and up-titration phase. Worsening renal function or hypotension usually can be improved after reduction in the dose of concomitantly administered diuretics, if possible. If renal function continues to deteriorate, however, lower doses of ACE inhibitors may need to be tried, or, in some cases, the ACE inhibitors may need to be discontinued. Patients who are unable to tolerate ACE inhibitors because of progressive renal dysfunction or other circulatory-renal limitations while on ACE inhibitors have a higher risk for mortality [71].

Gender and race

Most patients enrolled in the large randomized clinical trials that established the benefit of ACE inhibitors in patients who have LV systolic dysfunction were white men. Whether an equal effect is achieved in women and blacks has been controversial. There are several reasons to believe that certain subpopulations may not experience the same benefits as white men. There is evidence that ACE inhibitors exert a lesser effect on blood pressure in black compared with non-black hypertensive patients [72], and retrospective analyses have suggested that ACE inhibitors may not be as effective in black patients who have heart failure [73,74]. Similarly, men and women may respond differently to cardiac therapies. A preliminary analysis of one ACE inhibitor study suggested a trend toward lower mortality reduction in women compared with men [75]. A recent gender- and race-specific analysis of pooled data from seven large clinical trials, however, suggested that ACE inhibitors have survival benefit in women who have symptomatic heart failure and LV dysfunction, as well in black patients. Because of smaller numbers of these subgroups in the trials, definitive conclusions regarding the magnitude of the benefits compared with those seen in white males are not possible [76]. Pending the availability of more definitive data, however, current guidelines continue to recommend the use of ACE inhibition in women and black patients who have heart failure. Although clinical trials designed to address the issue of ACE inhibition in racial minorities may be desirable, a placebo-controlled trial would be unethical at this juncture. Finally, ethnic minorities such as blacks are genetically inhomogeneous populations, and data from subgroup analyses of large trials should not be used to withhold this life-saving treatment.

Summary

Based on overwhelming data demonstrating reduced morbidity and mortality, ACE inhibitors are a mainstay of therapy in patients with symptomatic and asymptomatic LV systolic dysfunction. Furthermore, ACE inhibitors may be beneficial in the prevention of heart failure in patients with high-risk cardiovascular profiles. Limited data suggest that they may also have some role in symptomatic patients with heart failure and preserved LVEF. Although ACE inhibitors likely exert a class effect, it is recommended that ACE inhibitors that reduced morbidity and mortality in clinical trials (eg, captopril, enalapril, lisinopril, and ramipril) be used preferentially because studies have defined clearly a dose for these agents that is effective in modifying the natural history of the disease. Attempts should be made to up-titrate patients to target doses of ACE inhibitors that have been used in clinical trials, if tolerated.

References

[1] Schrier RW, Abraham WT. Hormones and hemodynamics in heart failure. N Engl J Med 1999;341(8): 577–85.

[2] Folkow B, Johansson B, Mellander S. The comparative effects of angiotensin and noradrenaline on consecutive vascular sections. Acta Physiol Scand 1961;53:99–104.

[3] Zimmerman BG, Sybertz EJ, Wong PC. Interaction between sympathetic and renin-angiotensin system. J Hypertens 1984;2(6):581–7.

[4] Weber KT. Aldosterone in congestive heart failure. N Engl J Med 2001;345(23):1689–97.

[5] Padfield PL, Morton JJ. Effects of angiotensin II on arginine-vasopressin in physiological and pathological situations in man. J Endocrinol 1977;74(2): 251–9.

[6] Williams B. Angiotensin II and the pathophysiology of cardiovascular remodeling. Am J Cardiol 2001; 87(8A):10C–7C.

[7] Brown NJ, Vaughan DE. Angiotensin-converting enzyme inhibitors. Circulation 1998;97(14):1411–20.

[8] Sadoshima J, Izumo S. Molecular characterization of angiotensin II–induced hypertrophy of cardiac myocytes and hyperplasia of cardiac fibroblasts. Critical role of the AT1 receptor subtype. Circ Res 1993;73:413–23.

[9] Greenberg BH. Effects of angiotensin converting enzyme inhibitors on remodeling in clinical trials. J Card Fail 2002;8(6 Suppl):S486–90.

[10] Gavras I. Bradykinin-mediated effects of ACE inhibition. Kidney Int 1992;42(4):1020–9.

[11] Stein JH, Congbalay RC, Karsh DL, et al. The effect of bradykinin on proximal tubular sodium reabsorption in the dog: evidence for functional nephron heterogeneity. J Clin Invest 1972;51(7):1709–21.

[12] Gainer JV, Morrow JD, Loveland A, et al. Effect of bradykinin-receptor blockade on the response to angiotensin-converting-enzyme inhibitor in normotensive and hypertensive subjects. N Engl J Med 1998; 339(18):1285–92.

[13] McDonald KM, Mock J, d'Aloia A, et al. Bradykinin antagonism inhibits the antigrowth effect of converting enzyme inhibition in the dog myocardium after discrete transmural myocardial necrosis. Circulation 1995;91(7):2043–8.

[14] Antonaccio MJ. Development and pharmacology of angiotensin converting enzyme inhibitors. J Pharmacol 1983;14(Suppl 3):29–45.

[15] Ader R, Chatterjee K, Ports T, et al. Immediate and sustained hemodynamic and clinical improvement in chronic heart failure by an oral angiotensin-converting enzyme inhibitor. Circulation 1980;61(5):931–7.

[16] DiCarlo L, Chatterjee K, Parmley WW, et al. Enalapril: a new angiotensin-converting enzyme inhibitor in chronic heart failure: acute and chronic hemodynamic evaluations. J Am Coll Cardiol 1983;2(5):865–71.

[17] Chatterjee K, Parmley WW, Cohn JN, et al. A cooperative multicenter study of captopril in congestive heart failure: hemodynamic effects and long-term response. Am Heart J 1985;110(2):439–47.

[18] Pfeffer JM, Pfeffer MA, Braunwald E. Influence of chronic captopril therapy on the infarcted left ventricle of the rat. Circ Res 1985;57:84–95.

[19] O'Keefe JH, Wetzel M, Moe RR, et al. Should an angiotensin-converting enzyme inhibitor be standard therapy for patients with atherosclerotic disease? J Am Coll Cardiol 2001;37(1):1–8.

[20] Banerjee A, Talreja A, Sonnenblick EH, et al. Evolving rationale for angiotensin-converting enzyme inhibition in chronic heart failure. Mt Sinai J Med 2003;70(4):225–31.

[21] Garg R, Yusuf S. Overview of randomized trials of angiotensin-converting enzyme inhibitors on mortality and morbidity in patients with heart failure. JAMA 1995;273:1450–6.

[22] CONSENSUS Trial Study Group. Effects of enalapril on mortality in severe congestive heart failure:

results of the Cooperative North Scandanavian Ena-lapril Survival Study. N Engl J Med 1987;316: 1429–35.

[23] The SOLVD Investigators. Effect of enalapril on survival in patients with reduced left ventricular ejec-tion fractions and congestive heart failure. N Engl J Med 1991;325:293–302.

[24] Cohn JN, Johnson G, Ziesche S, et al. A comparison of enalapril with hydralazine-isosorbide dinitrate in the treatment of chronic congestive heart failure. N Engl J Med 1991;325:303–10.

[25] Narang R, Swedberg K, Cleland JG. What is the ideal study design for evaluation of treatment for heart failure? Insights from trials assessing the effect of ACE inhibitors on exercise capacity. Eur Heart J 1996;17(1):120–34.

[26] Cleland JG, Tendera M, Adamus J, et al. The peri-ndopril in elderly people with chronic heart failure (PEP-CHF) study. Eur Heart J 2006;27(19): 2338–45.

[27] Wang TJ, Evans JC, Benjamin EJ, et al. Natural his-tory of asymptomatic left ventricular systolic dys-function in the community. Circulation 2003; 108(8):977–82.

[28] Francis GS, Benedict C, Johnstone DE, et al. Com-parison of neuroendocrine activation in patients with left ventricular dysfunction with and without congestive heart failure A substudy of the Studies of Left Ventricular Dysfunction (SOLVD). Circula-tion 1990;82(5):1724–9.

[29] Kirlin PC, Grekin R, Das S, et al. Neurohumoral ac-tivation during exercise in congestive heart failure. Am J Med 1986;81(4):623–9.

[30] The SOLVD Investigators. Effect of enalapril on mortality and the development of heart failure in asymptomatic patients with reduced left ventricular ejection fractions. N Engl J Med 1992;327(10): 685–91.

[31] Konstam MA, Kronenberg MW, Rousseau MF, et al. Effects of the angiotensin converting enzyme inhibitor enalapril on the long-term progression of left ventricular dilatation in patients with asymp-tomatic systolic dysfunction. SOLVD (Studies of Left Ventricular Dysfunction) Investigators. Circu-lation 1993;88(5 Pt 1):2277–83.

[32] Pfeffer MA, Braunwald E, Moye LA, et al. Effect of captopril on mortality and morbidity in patients with left ventricular dysfunction after myocardial infarction. Results of the survival and ventricular enlargement trial. The SAVE Investigators. N Engl J Med 1992;327(10):669–77.

[33] Stadius ML, Davis K, Maynard C, et al. Risk strat-ification for 1 year survival based on characteristics identified in the early hours of acute myocardial infarction. The Western Washington Intra-coronary Streptokinase Trial. Circulation 1986; 74(4):703–11.

[34] White HD, Norris RM, Brown MA, et al. Left ventricular end-systolic volume as the major determinant of survival after recovery from myocar-dial infarction. Circulation 1987;76(1):44–51.

[35] McKay RG, Pfeffer MA, Pasternak RC, et al. Left ventricular remodeling after myocardial infarction: a corollary to infarct expansion. Circulation 1986; 74(4):693–702.

[36] Gaudron P, Eilles C, Ertl G, et al. Early remodelling of the left ventricle in patients with myocardial in-farction. Eur Heart J 1990;11(Suppl B):139–46.

[37] Pfeffer MA, Braunwald E. Ventricular remodeling after myocardial infarction. Experimental observa-tions and clinical implications. Circulation 1990; 81(4):1161–72.

[38] Pfeffer MA, Lamas GA, Vaughan DE, et al. Effect of captopril on progressive ventricular dilatation after anterior myocardial infarction. N Engl J Med 1988;319:80–6.

[39] Sharpe N, Murphy J, Smith H, et al. Treatment of patients with symptomless left ventricular dysfunc-tion after myocardial infarction. Lancet 1988; 1(8580):255–9.

[40] Kober L, Torp-Pedersen C, Carlsen JE, et al. A clin-ical trial of the angiotensin-converting-enzyme in-hibitor trandolapril in patients with left ventricular dysfunction after myocardial infarction. Trandolap-ril Cardiac Evaluation (TRACE) Study Group. N Engl J Med 1995;333(25):1670–6.

[41] AIRE Study. Effect of ramipril on mortality and morbidity of survivors of acute myocardial infarc-tion with clinical evidence of heart failure. Lancet 1993;342:821–8.

[42] Flather MD, Yusuf S, Kober L, et al. Long-term ACE-inhibitor therapy in patients with heart failure or left- ventricular dysfunction: a systematic over-view of data from individual patients. ACE-Inhibi-tor Myocardial Infarction Collaborative Group. Lancet 2000;355(9215):1575–81.

[43] Torp-Pedersen C, Kober L. Effect of ACE inhibitor trandolapril on life expectancy of patients with reduced left-ventricular function after acute myocardial infarction. TRACE Study Group. Tran-dolapril Cardiac Evaluation. Lancet 1999; 354(9172):9–12.

[44] Hall AS, Murray GD, Ball SG. Follow-up study of patients randomly allocated ramipril or placebo for heart failure after acute myocardial infarction: AIRE Extension (AIREX) Study Acute Infarction Ramipril Efficacy. Lancet 1997;349(9064):1493–7.

[45] Brilla CG, Funck RC, Rupp H. Lisinopril-mediated regression of myocardial fibrosis in patients with hy-pertensive heart disease. Circulation 2000;102(12): 1388–93.

[46] Weber KT, Brilla CG. Pathological hypertrophy and cardiac interstitium. Fibrosis and renin-angio-tensin-aldosterone system. Circulation 1991;83(6): 1849–65.

[47] Angeli F, Verdecchia P, Reboldi GP, et al. Meta-analysis of effectiveness or lack thereof of angioten-sin-converting enzyme inhibitors for prevention of

heart failure in patients with systemic hypertension. Am J Cardiol 2004;93(2):240–3.

[48] Mills E, Montori VM, Thabane L. Angiotensin-converting enzyme inhibitor meta-analysis provides misleading conclusion. Am J Cardiol 2004;94(1): 149.

[49] Yusuf S, Sleight P, Pogue J, et al. Effects of an angiotensin-converting-enzyme inhibitor, ramipril, on cardiovascular events in high-risk patients. The Heart Outcomes Prevention Evaluation Study Investigators. N Engl J Med 2000;342(3):145–53.

[50] Arnold JM, Yusuf S, Young J, et al. Prevention of heart failure in patients in the Heart Outcomes Prevention Evaluation (HOPE) study. Circulation 2003;107(9):1284–90.

[51] Dagenais GR, Pogue J, Fox K, et al. Angiotensin-converting enzyme inhibitors in stable vascular disease without left ventricular systolic dysfunction or heart failure: a combined analysis of three trials. Lancet 2006;368(9535):581–8.

[52] Hunt SA, Abraham WT, Chin MH, et al. ACC/AHA 2005 guideline update for the diagnosis and management of chronic heart failure in the adult: a report of the American College of Cardiology/American Heart Association Task Force on Practice Guidelines. J Am Coll Cardiol 2005;46(6): e1–e82.

[53] Packer M. Do angiotensin-converting enzyme inhibitors prolong life in patients with heart failure treated in clinical practice. J Am Coll Cardiol 1996;28:1323–7.

[54] Ljungman S, Kjekshus J, Swedberg K. Renal function in severe congestive heart failure during treatment with enalapril (the Cooperative North Scandinavian Enalapril Survival Study [CONSENSUS] Trial). Am J Cardiol 1992;70(4):479–87.

[55] Massie BM, Kramer BL, Topic N. Lack of relationship between the short-term hemodynamic effects of captopril and subsequent clinical responses. Circulation 1984;69(6):1135–41.

[56] Chen YT, Wang Y, Radford MJ, et al. Angiotensin-converting enzyme inhibitor dosages in elderly patients with heart failure. Am Heart J 2001;141(3): 410–7.

[57] Pacher R, Stanek B, Globits S, et al. Effects of two different enalapril dosages on clinical, haemodynamic, and neurohumoral response of patients with severe congestive heart failure. Eur Heart J 1996;17(8):1223–32.

[58] Uretsky BF, Shaver JA, Liang CS, et al. Modulation of hemodynamic effects with a converting enzyme inhibitor: acute hemodynamic dose-response relationship of a new angiotensin converting enzyme inhibitor, lisinopril, with observations on long-term clinical, functional, and biochemical responses. Am Heart J 1988;116(2 Pt 1):480–8.

[59] Riegger GA. Effects of quinapril on exercise tolerance in patients with mild to moderate heart failure. Eur Heart J 1991;12(6):705–11.

[60] Wollert KC, Studer R, von Bulow B, et al. Survival after myocardial infarction in the rat. Role of tissue angiotensin-converting enzyme inhibition. Circulation 1994;90:2457–67.

[61] Tang WH, Vagelos RH, Yee YG, et al. Neurohormonal and clinical responses to high- versus low-dose enalapril therapy in chronic heart failure. J Am Coll Cardiol 2002;39(1):70–8.

[62] Clinical outcome with enalapril in symptomatic chronic heart failure; a dose comparison. The NETWORK Investigators. Eur Heart J 1998;19(3): 481–9.

[63] Nanas JN, Alexopoulos G, Anastasiou-Nana MI, et al. Outcome of patients with congestive heart failure treated with standard versus high doses of enalapril: a multicenter study. High Enalapril Dose Study Group. J Am Coll Cardiol 2000;36(7):2090–5.

[64] Williams SG, Cooke GA, Wright DJ, et al. Disparate results of ACE inhibitor dosage on exercise capacity in heart failure: a reappraisal of vasodilator therapy and study design. Int J Cardiol 2001; 77(2–3):239–45.

[65] Packer M, Poole-Wilson PA, Armstrong PW, et al. Comparative effects of low and high doses of the angiotensin-converting enzyme inhibitor, lisinopril, on morbidity and mortality in chronic heart failure. ATLAS Study Group. Circulation 1999;100(23): 2312–8.

[66] Zannad F, van den Broek SA, Bory M. Comparison of treatment with lisinopril versus enalapril for congestive heart failure. Am J Cardiol 1992;70(10): 78C–83C.

[67] Packer M, Medina N, Yushak M. Relation between serum sodium concentration and the hemodynamic and clinical responses to converting enzyme inhibition with captopril in severe heart failure. J Am Coll Cardiol 1984;3(4):1035–43.

[68] Dries DL, Exner DV, Domanski MJ, et al. The prognostic implications of renal insufficiency in asymptomatic and symptomatic patients with left ventricular systolic dysfunction. J Am Coll Cardiol 2000,35(3).681–9.

[69] McAlister FA, Ezekowitz J, Tonelli M, et al. Renal insufficiency and heart failure: prognostic and therapeutic implications from a prospective cohort study. Circulation 2004;109(8):1004–9.

[70] Knight EL, Glynn RJ, McIntyre KM, et al. Predictors of decreased renal function in patients with heart failure during angiotensin-converting enzyme inhibitor therapy: results from the studies of left ventricular dysfunction (SOLVD). Am Heart J 1999; 138(5 Pt 1):849–55.

[71] Kittleson M, Hurwitz S, Shah MR, et al. Development of circulatory-renal limitations to angiotensin-converting enzyme inhibitors identifies patients with severe heart failure and early mortality. J Am Coll Cardiol 2003;41(11):2029–35.

[72] Materson BJ, Reda DJ, Cushman WC, et al. Single-drug therapy for hypertension in men. A comparison

of six antihypertensive agents with placebo. The Department of Veterans Affairs Cooperative Study Group on Antihypertensive Agents. N Engl J Med 1993;328(13):914–21.

[73] Vasan RS, Benjamin EJ, Levy D. Congestive heart failure with normal left ventricular systolic function. Clinical approaches to the diagnosis and treatment of diastolic heart failure. Arch Intern Med 1996; 156(2):146–57.

[74] Carson P, Ziesche S, Johnson G, et al. Racial differences in response to therapy for heart failure: analysis of the vasodilator-heart failure trials. Vasodilator-Heart Failure Trial Study Group. J Card Fail 1999;5(3):178–87.

[75] Limacher MC, Yusuf S, for the SOLVD Investigators. Gender differences in the Studies of Left Ventricular Dysfunction (SOLVD): a preliminary report. In: Wenger NK, Sperof L, Packard B, editors. Cardiovascular health and disease and women. Greenwich (CT): Le Jaq Communications; 1993. p. 345–8.

[76] Shekelle PG, Rich MW, Morton SC, et al. Efficacy of angiotensin-converting enzyme inhibitors and beta-blockers in the management of left ventricular systolic dysfunction according to race, gender, and diabetic status: a meta-analysis of major clinical trials. J Am Coll Cardiol 2003;41(9):1529–38.

[77] Jong P, Yusuf S, Rousseau MF, et al. Effect of enalapril on 12-year survival and life expectancy in patients with left ventricular systolic dysfunction: a follow-up study. Lancet 2003;361(9372): 1843–8.

Aldosterone Blockade in Patients with Chronic Heart Failure

Bertram Pitt, MD

University of Michigan School of Medicine, 1500 East Medical Center Drive, Ann Arbor, MI 48109, USA

Aldosterone has long been recognized as being important for sodium retention and volume control. Angiotensin-converting enzyme inhibitors (ACE-Is) and angiotensin receptor blocking agents (ARBs) were once believed to prevent the production of aldosterone from the adrenal gland. However, despite the use of ACE-Is or ARBs in the Randomized Evaluation of Strategies for Left Ventricular Dysfunction (RESOLVD) trial [1], aldosterone levels were only transiently reduced.

Although angiotensin II (ATII), through stimulation of the AT1 receptor, is an important stimulus for aldosterone production, other stimuli have been shown to be important in certain circumstances. For example, a change in serum sodium levels in the angiotensinogen-knockout mouse, which has no ATII, causes aldosterone levels to increase [2]. Thus, despite the use of an ACE-I or ARB, aldosterone production from the adrenal gland cannot be blocked.

Aldosterone has also been found to be far more important in the pathophysiology of cardiovascular disease than originally believed. A clue to the importance of aldosterone in cardiovascular disease can be found when comparing patients who have primary aldosteronism with those who have essential hypertension at equal blood pressures. Patients who have primary aldosteronism have been shown to have significantly increased incidence of left ventricular hypertrophy, atrial fibrillation, myocardial infarction (MI), and stroke [3]. Patients who have primary aldosteronism have also been shown to have a significant decrease in pancreatic β-cell function, an increase in serum glucose, and insulin resistance [4,5], suggesting that aldosterone plays an important role in the metabolic syndrome. The importance of aldosterone in the pathophysiology of cardiovascular disease can also be seen from the results of the Randomized Aldactone Evaluation Study (RALES trial), which showed that aldosterone blockade in patients who had severe heart failure from systolic left ventricular dysfunction (SLVD) caused significantly reduced morbidity and mortality [6].

Aldosterone blockade with spironolactone 12.5 to 50 mg/d has been shown to reduce total mortality by 30% and hospitalization in patients who have severe heart failure (New York Heart Association [NYHA] class III–IV) and a history of class IV heart failure because of SLVD [6]. These beneficial effects were seen in men and women; patients who had ischemic and nonischemic cardiomyopathy; patients who had diabetes mellitus and those who did not; and young and elderly individuals. In the RALES trials, almost all patients were treated with an ACE-I or ARB and a loop diuretic, but only 10% to 11% were taking a β-adrenergic–receptor blocking agent (BB), because RALES was designed before the Carvedilol Prospective Randomized Cumulative Survival (COPERNICUS) trial showed the effectiveness of BBs in patients who had severe heart failure caused by SLVD [7]. However, the point estimate of benefit for spironolactone tended to be even greater in patients not treated with a BB compared with those who were. Subsequent studies have shown that aldosterone blockade is effective in reducing total mortality in patients post-MI complicated by SLVD and clinical heart failure [8] treated with a BB and an ACE-I or ARB.

The American College of Cardiology/American Heart Association and European Society of Cardiology guidelines recognize aldosterone

---

E-mail address: bpitt@umich.edu

blockade as a class 1 indication for patients who have severe heart failure caused by SLVD [9,10]. However, patients who have a serum potassium (K+) level greater than 5.0 meq/L or a serum creatinine level greater than 2.5 mg/dL were excluded from RALES [6]. In RALES [6], patients were randomized to receive either 25 mg/d of spironolactone or placebo, and the serum K+ was frequently monitored. The dose of study drug could be down-titrated to 25 mg every other day at any time if the serum potassium was 5.5 meq/L or higher, and the drug discontinued if the serum K+ was greater than 6.0 meq/L. The dose of study drug could also be up-titrated to 50 mg/d after 1 month if evidence was seen of progressive heart failure. Serum K+ should be measured whenever a change in electrolyte status is suspected, such as after an episode of frequent vomiting or diarrhea, and whenever a drug affecting K+ excretion is added, such as a nonsteroidal anti-inflammatory drug (NSAID) or Cox-2 inhibitor. Although an increase occurred in the incidence of serious hyperkalemia (K+ >6.0 meq/L) in patients randomized to spironolactone in RALES [6], no deaths were attributable to hyperkalemia in patients randomized to spironolactone, and total mortality was significantly reduced.

However, since the RALES results [6] were published, several reports have suggested that the clinical practice use of spironolactone in patients who have heart failure is associated with a high incidence of serious hyperkalemia, resulting in increased hospitalization and occasionally renal failure, the need for dialysis, and death [11–14]. A critical review of these publications shows that higher doses of spironolactone than those used in RALES were often administered, often to patients who had a serum creatinine level greater than 2.5 mg/dL or a serum K+ level greater than 5.0 meq/L, without monitoring serum K+ or adjusting the dose of spironolactone according to the level of serum K+. For example, one study in which patients were given spironolactone for heart failure showed a 15% incidence of serious hyperkalemia [15]. However, approximately one third of the patients in this study did not have a single measurement of serum K+. It would be considered malpractice if a patient who had atrial fibrillation experienced a major bleeding episode without a single determination of their international normalized ratio or other index of coagulation. Similarly, to benefit from the effects of aldosterone blockade in reducing mortality in patients who have heart failure caused by SLVD,

serum K+ must be monitored and aldosterone blockade dose adjusted accordingly. Furthermore, in patients who have heart failure, the optimum level of serum K+ has been suggested to be between 4.0 and 5.5 meq/L. Spironolactone should not be discontinued in a patient who has heart failure with a serum K+ of 5.5 meq/L, but the dose should be reduced by half and the serum K+ closely monitored and discontinued if the serum K+ is 6.0 meq/L or higher. Additionally, because the serum creatinine level may underestimate the extent of renal dysfunction in elderly patients, determining the estimated glomerular filtration rate (eGFR) before considering the use of an aldosterone blockade would be prudent. Aldosterone blockade is contraindicated in patients who have an eGFR less than 30 mL/min. Patients who have an eGFR between 30 and 60 mL/min should be closely monitored for changes in serum K+, and drugs that could result in K+ retention, such as NSAIDs, should be avoided if possible.

Further support for the use of aldosterone blockades in patients who have heart failure is provided by the results of the Eplerenone Post-Acute Myocardial Infarction Heart Failure Efficacy and Survival Study (EPHESUS trial) [8], in which patients who had evidence of SLVD and heart failure post-MI were randomized to receive the aldosterone blockade eplerenone 25 to 50 mg/d or placebo between 3 and 14 days post-MI. Eplerenone is more selective for the mineralocorticoid receptor compared with spironolactone, which also affects androgen and progesterone receptors resulting in breast pain and gynecomastia in men and menstrual irregularities in premenopausal women. Approximately 50 mg of eplerenone is equivalent to 25 mg of spironolactone. In the EPHESUS trial [8], almost all patients were treated with an ACE-I or an ARB and three quarters with a BB. Patients generally underwent contemporary therapy, including an aspirin, statin, and reperfusion. Patients randomized to receive eplerenone beginning at a dose of 25 mg, which could be up-titrated to 50 mg at 1 month, were found to have a 15% significant reduction in total mortality and a reduction in the coprimary end point of cardiovascular death/hospitalization for heart failure. A 21% reduction in sudden cardiac death was also seen.

Of particular interest was the finding that total mortality was significantly reduced by 31% and sudden cardiac death by 37% at 30 days post-randomization [16]. The results were even better in the subset of patients who had a left ventricular ejection fraction of 30% or less before randomization, with a reduction in total mortality by 43% and sudden cardiac death by 58% at 30 days post-randomization. This finding is important because the period of greatest risk in patients who have heart failure on admission is the first 30 days post-MI [17], and other strategies, such as the implantation of a defibrillator, have not been successful in reducing mortality when attempted during this period [18]. However, the mean time from onset of infarction to randomization was 7 days in EPHESUS [8], and therefore a mean of 30 days after randomization is actually 37 days post-MI.

A recent retrospective analysis of the EPHESUS data showed that patients randomized to eplerenone between day 3 and 7 had a significant reduction in total mortality, whereas those randomized to eplerenone more than 7 days post-MI did not experience a significant benefit [19]. Hayashi and colleagues [20] showed that when an aldosterone blockade is administered on day 1 post-MI to patients who had a first anterior MI undergoing primary percutaneous transluminal coronary angioplasty and is continued for 1 month, they experience a significant improvement in ventricular remodeling and myocardial collagen formation. The study by Hyashi and colleagues [20] and the recent finding that almost all mortality benefit from administering eplerenone post-MI in EPHESUS [8] occurred in those who received it less than 7 days from randomization suggest that an aldosterone blockade should be administered as early as possible in patients post-MI in whom it is indicated. When the EPHESUS [8] study was planned, there was no experience in using an aldosterone blockade early post-MI and it was feared that it might cause hypotension, which could lead to further ischemic damage. However, the results of the study by Hyashi and colleagues [20] and an analysis of the changes in blood pressure after administering eplerenone post-MI suggest that this strategy is safe and does not result in hypotension. In EPHESUS [8], patients were divided into quartiles according to their baseline systolic blood pressure. Patients in the lowest quartile of systolic blood pressure (mean 104 mm Hg) randomized to receive eplerenone had an increase in systolic blood pressure of approximately 6 mm Hg over the first week, similar to patients randomized to placebo, whereas patients in the highest quartile of systolic blood pressure (mean 147 mm Hg) had a 17 mmHg decline in systolic blood pressure similar to placebo [21]. This experience is different from that encountered when an ARB is added to an ACE-I post-MI, when a decline in blood pressure of several millimeters of mercury can be anticipated [22].

Although the mean blood pressure at randomization into EPHESUS [8] was normal, approximately two thirds of the patients had a history of hypertension. Almost all of the benefit of eplerenone in reducing total mortality and sudden cardiac death was found in those who had a history of hypertension [23]. Patients who did not have a history of hypertension showed a significant reduction in hospitalization for heart failure but not mortality. The explanation for this benefit in mortality compared with those who did not have a history of hypertension is uncertain, but is possibly related to the occurrence of left ventricular hypertrophy associated with an up-regulation of the mineralocorticoid receptor and an increase in calcium channel expression in those who have a history of hypertension. These findings, along with the finding that aldosterone blockade reduces left ventricular mass, myocardial collagen formation, and improves vascular compliance [24–26], have potential implications for the use of aldosterone blockade in patients who have hypertension before the onset of MI. The beneficial effects of eplerenone on total mortality shown in EPHESUS [8] have resulted in a class 1 indication for aldosterone blockade in patients who have SLVD and heart failure post-MI, and further support the use of aldosterone blockade in patients who have chronic severe heart failure because of SLVD, as studied in RALES [6].

However, many clinicians have been concerned about the increasing use of polypharmacy in patients who have chronic heart failure caused by SLVD and those who have heart failure post-MI, and have wondered whether the results of RALES and EPHESUS could result in the elimination of an ACE-I, ARB, or BB, or a change in their sequence of administration. Increasing evidence, however, has suggested that the combination of an ACE-I or ARB with an aldosterone blockade is more effective than either one alone for preventing ventricular remodeling [27]. Therefore, in a patient who has severe heart failure because of SLVD, it would be appropriate to institute therapy simultaneously with an ACE-I or ARB and an aldosterone blockade, providing renal function is adequate (eGFR >60 mL/min per 1.73 m^2) and the serum is less than 5.0 meq/L. In patients who have an eGFR greater than 30 but less than 60 mL/min per 1.73 m^2, it would be prudent to administer an ACE-I or ARB first, and an aldosterone blockade only to those whose renal function and serum potassium remain stable (eGFR >50 mL/min per 1.73 m^2 and serum K+ <5.0 meq/L).

The question as to whether an ARB should be first added to an ACE-I or aldosterone blockade in a patient who has severe heart failure caused by SLVD is difficult to answer, because no studies have compared these strategies. The addition of candesartan to an ACE-I in the Candesartan in Heart Failure: Assessment of Reduction in Mortality and Morbidity (CHARM)-Added trial was effective in reducing cardiovascular mortality/hospitalization for heart failure but not total mortality [28]. The reduction in total mortality in RALES [6] and EPHESUS [8] when an aldosterone blockade was added to an ACE-I or ARB would, in the author's opinion, favor first adding an aldosterone blockade to an ACE-I or ARB before the addition of an ARB to an ACE-I, or an ACE-I to an ARB is considered. However, further direct comparative studies are required to reach a definitive answer on the relative effectiveness of these two strategies. In a patient taking an ACE-I and ARB with evidence of progressive heart failure, adding an aldosterone blockade might be advantageous. Similarly, in a patient on an ACE-I and aldosterone blockade, an ARB could be added if renal function and serum potassium are stable. Although the experience with triple Renin Angiotensin Aldosterone System (RAAS) blockade is limited, several patients in CHARM-Added [28] on an ACE-I, ARB, and aldosterone blockade seemed to tolerate these agents. In the Aliskiren Observation of Heart Failure Treatment Study (ALOFT) [29], approximately one third of patients on an ACE-I or ARB, an aldosterone blockade, and a direct renin inhibitor seemed to tolerate and benefit from triple RAAS blockade.

The situation is different regarding the use of a BB relative to an aldosterone blockade when added to an ACE-I or ARB. Although the COPERNICUS trial [7] showed that BB was effective in reducing mortality in patients who had severe heart failure caused by SLVD, these patients were euvolemic. In patients who have severe heart failure caused by SLVD with evidence of volume overload, this author believes it would be prudent to add an aldosterone blockade to an ACE-I or ARB before considering adding a BB. Furthermore, aldosterone blockade has been

shown to prevent isoproterenol-induced myocardial damage and to prevent norepinephrine release from sympathetic nerve terminals [30,31]. The addition of an aldosterone blockade to an ACE-I or ARB should therefore provide protection against β-adrenergic–induced myocardial damage and improve the speed and tolerability of BB addition once the patient is euvolemic.

The use of an aldosterone blockade in patients who have mild (NYHA class II) heart failure is currently not indicated, because no large-scale randomized study has evaluated this strategy. However, in patients who have mild heart failure caused by SLVD maintained on an ACE-I or ARB and a BB, evidence shows that addition of an aldosterone blockade is associated with a beneficial effect on ventricular remodeling [32]. A large-scale, prospective, double-blind, randomized study of eplerenone in patients who have NYHA class II heart failure and SLVD is currently ongoing [33] and should show whether aldosterone blockade is effective in reducing cardiovascular mortality/hospitalization for heart failure. Aldosterone blockade has also been suggested to be of benefit in patients who have asymptomatic left ventricular dysfunction (ALVD). Costello-Boerrigter and colleagues [34] recently showed that DOCA, which is an agonist of the mineralocorticoid receptor, administered to a canine model results in the development of myocardial fibrosis. However, the kidneys retain their ability to excrete sodium during this early stage of heart failure. Therefore, the authors suggest that an aldosterone blockade administered at this early stage of left ventricular dysfunction in patients who have ALVD might play a role in stopping the progression of myocardial dysfunction before the onset of renal dysfunction and sodium retention, and the development of manifest heart failure with volume overload.

Aldosterone blockade may also be beneficial in patients who have heart failure and preserved or normal left ventricular function (HFnlEF), and has also been shown to improve vascular compliance [26]. In patients who had essential hypertension and left ventricular hypertrophy, eplerenone was shown to be as effective as the ACE-I enalapril in regressing left ventricular hypertrophy and reducing the incidence of albuminuria, whereas their combination was more effective than either alone [24]. In patients who had hypertension and diastolic heart failure, spironolactone was shown to significantly improve echocardiographic indices of diastolic function [35]. The role of aldosterone blockade in patients who have HFnlEF is currently being evaluated in a large-scale randomized study sponsored by the National Heart, Lung, and Blood Institute (Treatment of Preserved Cardiac Function Heart Failure with an Aldosterone Antagonist trial) [33]. Patients who had a history of heart failure and preserved systolic function after control of their blood pressure are being randomized to spironolactone beginning at a dose of 15 mg/d with up-titration to 45 mg/d or placebo if their serum potassium is less than 5.0 meq/L and their eGFR greater than 30 mL/min per 1.73 m^2. The primary end point of this study is cardiovascular mortality/hospitalization for heart failure. In the CHARM-Preserved trial, the use of candesartan was not effective in reducing cardiovascular mortality, although it reduced hospitalization for heart failure [36]. The role of an ARB in patients who have HFnlEF is currently being investigated in the IPRESERVE trial with the ARB irbesartan [37]. Regardless of the outcome, an aldosterone blockade added to an ACE-I or ARB can be expected to be effective in improving diastolic left ventricular function and cardiovascular events in these patients.

The mechanisms through which aldosterone blockade is effective in reducing total mortality in patients who have severe heart failure because of SLVD and those who have heart failure and SLVD post-MI were mentioned earlier. Aldosterone production from the adrenal gland cannot be prevented by an ACE-I or ARB, and aldosterone, although important for sodium retention and volume control, has also been shown to be an independent risk factor for MI, stroke, atrial fibrillation, and left ventricular hypertrophy [3]. As importantly, an increase in mineralocorticoid receptor expression occurs in heart failure [38], as does an increase in the serum concentration of aldosterone associated with an increase in myocardial calcium channel expression [39], which would predispose to ventricular arrhythmias and sudden cardiac death. In a model of heart failure post-MI, an early prolongation of the ventricular action potential was found, along with an increase in myocardial calcium concentration [40]. The administration of an aldosterone blockade significantly reversed these changes, which may account for its beneficial effect on sudden cardiac death. Aldosterone blockade has also been shown to prevent myocardial fibrosis and ventricular remodeling [20,32], which could account for their beneficial effects in preventing hospitalization for heart failure and death from progressive heart failure. In addition, aldosterone blockade have been shown to improve antioxidant reserves through increasing the availability of the enzyme G6PD [41]; increase the availability of nitric oxide; improve endothelial function; and prevent experimental atherosclerosis [42–46]. Aldosterone blockade has also been shown to decrease ACE and AT1 receptor expression [47], all of which would tend to improve vasodilatation and prevent the adverse effects of ATII on the cardiovascular system.

Summary

Aldosterone blockade has been shown to be effective in reducing mortality in patients who have severe heart failure because of SLVD and those who have heart failure and SLVD post-MI [6,8]. However, based on the mechanisms described in this article, aldosterone blockade may also be beneficial in patients who have NYHA class II heart failure, ALVD, and HFnlEF. Considering the beneficial effects of aldosterone blockade on improving nitric oxide availability, endothelial function, and atherosclerosis, it can also be postulated that an aldosterone blockade would add to the benefits of an ACE-I in patients who have coronary artery disease, such as those in the HOPE study [48]. However, these hypotheses must be confirmed in well-designed, large-scale, prospectively randomized studies.

References

[1] McKelvie RS, Yusuf S, Pericak D, et al. Comparison of candesartan, enalapril, and their combination in congestive heart failure: randomized evaluation of strategies for left ventricular dysfunction (RESOLVD) pilot study. The RESOLVD Pilot Study Investigators. Circulation 1999;100(10): 1056–64.

[2] Okubo S, Niimura F, Nishimura H, et al. Angiotensin-independent mechanism for aldosterone synthesis during chronic extracellular fluid volume depletion. J Clin Invest 1997;99(5):855–60.

[3] Milliez P, Deangelis N, Rucker-Martin C, et al. Spironolactone reduces fibrosis of dilated atria during heart failure in rats with myocardial infarction. Eur Heart J 2005;26(20):2193–9.

[4] Mosso LM, Carvajal CA, Maiz A, et al. A possible association between primary aldosteronism and a lower beta-cell function. J Hypertens 2007; 25(10):2125–30.

[5] Hitomi H, Kiyomoto H, Nishiyama A, et al. Aldosterone suppresses insulin signaling via the

downregulation of insulin receptor substrate-1 in vascular smooth muscle cells. Hypertension 2007; 50(4):750–5.

[6] Pitt B, Zannad F, Remme WJ, et al. The effect of spironolactone on morbidity and mortality in patients with severe heart failure. Randomized Aldactone Evaluation Study Investigators. N Engl J Med 1999;341(10):709–17.

[7] Packer M, Coats AJ, Fowler MB, et al. Effect of carvedilol on survival in severe chronic heart failure. N Engl J Med 2001;344(22):1651–8.

[8] Pitt B, Remme W, Zannad F, et al. Eplerenone, a selective aldosterone blocker, in patients with left ventricular dysfunction after myocardial infarction. N Engl J Med 2003;348(14):1309–21.

[9] Hunt SA. ACC/AHA 2005 guideline update for the diagnosis and management of chronic heart failure in the adult: a report of the American College of Cardiology/American Heart Association Task Force on Practice Guidelines (Writing Committee to Update the 2001 Guidelines for the Evaluation and Management of Heart Failure). J Am Coll Cardiol 2005; 46(6):e1–82.

[10] Nieminen MS, Bohm M, Cowie MR, et al. Executive summary of the guidelines on the diagnosis and treatment of acute heart failure: the Task Force on Acute Heart Failure of the European Society of Cardiology. Eur Heart J 2005;26(4):384–416.

[11] Berry C, McMurray JJ. Serious adverse events experienced by patients with chronic heart failure taking spironolactone. Heart 2001;85(4):E8.

[12] Schepkens H, Vanholder R, Billiouw JM, et al. Life-threatening hyperkalemia during combined therapy with angiotensin-converting enzyme inhibitors and spironolactone: an analysis of 25 cases. Am J Med 2001;110(6):438–41.

[13] Svensson M, Gustafsson F, Galatius S, et al. Hyperkalaemia and impaired renal function in patients taking spironolactone for congestive heart failure: retrospective study. BMJ 2003;327(7424): 1141–2.

[14] Juurlink DN, Mamdani MM, Lee DS, et al. Rates of hyperkalemia after publication of the Randomized Aldactone Evaluation Study. N Engl J Med 2004; 351(6):543–51.

[15] Shah KB, Rao K, Sawyer R, et al. The adequacy of laboratory monitoring in patients treated with spironolactone for congestive heart failure. J Am Coll Cardiol 2005;46(5):845–9.

[16] Pitt B, White H, Nicolau J, et al. Eplerenone reduces mortality 30 days after randomization following acute myocardial infarction in patients with left ventricular systolic dysfunction and heart failure. J Am Coll Cardiol 2005;46(3):425–31.

[17] Steg PG, Dabbous OH, Feldman LJ, et al. Determinants and prognostic impact of heart failure complicating acute coronary syndromes: observations from the Global Registry of Acute Coronary Events (GRACE). Circulation 2004;109(4):494–9.

[18] Holnloser S, Kuck K, Dorian P, et al. The DINAMIT investigators. Prophylactic use of an implantable cardioverter-defibrillator after acute myocardial infarction. N Engl J Med 2004;351:2481–8.

[19] Zannad, Adamopoulos, Fay, et al. P484: how early should eplerenone be initiated in acute myocardial infarction complicated by heart failure? An analysis of early vs. initiation in the EPHESUS trial [abstract]. Eur Heart J 2007;28:52.

[20] Hayashi M, Tsutamoto T, Wada A, et al. Immediate administration of mineralocorticoid receptor antagonist spironolactone prevents post-infarct left ventricular remodeling associated with suppression of a marker of myocardial collagen synthesis in patients with first anterior acute myocardial infarction. Circulation 2003;107(20):2559–65.

[21] Banas J, Krum H, Corbalan R, et al. Impact of eplerenone on blood pressure in post-acute myocardial infarction patients with heart failure and left ventricular systolic dysfunction: results from EPHESUS. Submitted for publication.

[22] Pfeffer MA, McMurray JJ, Velazquez EJ, et al. Valsartan, captopril, or both in myocardial infarction complicated by heart failure, left ventricular dysfunction, or both. N Engl J Med 2003;349(20): 1893–906.

[23] Pitt B, Krum H, Nicolau J, et al. The EPHESUS trial: effect of eplerenone in patients with a baseline history of hypertension. Circulation 2003;108 (Suppl):599.

[24] Pitt B, Reichek N, Willenbrock R, et al. Effects of eplerenone, enalapril, and eplerenone/enalapril in patients with essential hypertension and left ventricular hypertrophy: the 4E-left ventricular hypertrophy study. Circulation 2003;108(15):1831–8.

[25] Zannad F, Alla F, Dousset B, et al. Limitation of excessive extracellular matrix turnover may contribute to survival benefit of spironolactone therapy in patients with congestive heart failure: insights from the randomized aldactone evaluation study (RALES). Rales Investigators. Circulation 2000; 102(22):2700–6.

[26] Lacolley P, Labat C, Pujol A, et al. Increased carotid wall elastic modulus and fibronectin in aldosterone-salt-treated rats: effects of eplerenone. Circulation 2002;106(22):2848–53.

[27] Fraccarollo D, Galuppo P, Hildemann S, et al. Additive improvement of left ventricular remodeling and neurohormonal activation by aldosterone receptor blockade with eplerenone and ACE inhibition in rats with myocardial infarction. J Am Coll Cardiol 2003;42(9):1666–73.

[28] McMurray J, Pitt B, Latini R. Effects of the oral direct renin inhibitor aliskiren in patients with symptomatic heart failure. To be presented at the ESC 9/2007. Lancet, in press.

[29] Pitt B, McMurray J, Latini R, et al. Neurohumoral effects of a new oral direct renin inhibitor in stable heart failure: the Aliskiren Observation of Heart

Failure Treatment Study (ALOFT). Circulation 2007;116(16):II–549.

[30] Kasama S, Toyama T, Kumakura H, et al. Effect of spironolactone on cardiac sympathetic nerve activity and left ventricular remodeling in patients with dilated cardiomyopathy. J Am Coll Cardiol 2003; 41(4):574–81.

[31] Cittadini A, Monti MG, Isgaard J, et al. Aldosterone receptor blockade improves left ventricular remodeling and increases ventricular fibrillation threshold in experimental heart failure. Cardiovasc Res 2003;58(3):555–64.

[32] Chan AK, Sanderson JE, Wang T, et al. Aldosterone receptor antagonism induces reverse remodeling when added to angiotensin receptor blockade in chronic heart failure. J Am Coll Cardiol 2007; 50(7):591–6.

[33] Aldosterone antagonist therapy for adults with heart failure and preserved systolic function. Available at: http://www.clinicaltrials.gov. 2007.

[34] Costello-Boerrigter LC, Boerrigter G, Harty GJ, et al. Mineralocorticoid escape by the kidney but not the heart in experimental asymptomatic left ventricular dysfunction. Hypertension 2007;50(3):481–8.

[35] Mottram PM, Haluska B, Leano R, et al. Effect of aldosterone antagonism on myocardial dysfunction in hypertensive patients with diastolic heart failure. Circulation 2004;110(5):558–65.

[36] Yusuf S, Pfeffer MA, Swedberg K, et al. Effects of candesartan in patients with chronic heart failure and preserved left-ventricular ejection fraction: the CHARM-Preserved Trial. Lancet 2003;362(9386): 777–81.

[37] Carson P, Massie BM, McKelvie R, et al. The irbesartan in heart failure with preserved systolic function (I-PRESERVE) trial: rationale and design. J Card Fail 2005;11(8):576–85.

[38] Yoshida M, Ma J, Tomita T, et al. Mineralocorticoid receptor is overexpressed in cardiomyocytes of patients with congestive heart failure. Congest Heart Fail 2005;11(1):12–6.

[39] Lalevee N, Rebsamen MC, Barrere-Lemaire S, et al. Aldosterone increases T-type calcium channel expression and in vitro beating frequency in neonatal rat cardiomyocytes. Cardiovasc Res 2005;67(2): 216–24.

[40] Perrier E, Kerfant BG, Lalevee N, et al. Mineralocorticoid receptor antagonism prevents the electrical remodeling that precedes cellular hypertrophy after myocardial infarction. Circulation 2004;110(7): 776–83.

[41] Leopold JA, Dam A, Maron BA, et al. Aldosterone impairs vascular reactivity by decreasing glucose-6-phosphate dehydrogenase activity. Nat Med 2007; 13(2):189–97.

[42] Kobayashi N, Yoshida K, Nakano S, et al. Cardioprotective mechanisms of eplerenone on cardiac performance and remodeling in failing rat hearts. Hypertension 2006;47(4):671–9.

[43] Bauersachs J, Heck M, Fraccarollo D, et al. Addition of spironolactone to angiotensin-converting enzyme inhibition in heart failure improves endothelial vasomotor dysfunction: role of vascular superoxide anion formation and endothelial nitric oxide synthase expression. J Am Coll Cardiol 2002;39(2): 351–8.

[44] Rajagopalan S, Duquaine D, King S, et al. Mineralocorticoid receptor antagonism in experimental atherosclerosis. Circulation 2002;105(18):2212–6.

[45] Struthers A. Impact of aldosterone on vascular pathophysiology. Congest Heart Fail 2002;8:18–22.

[46] Takai S, Jin D, Muramatsu M, et al. Eplerenone inhibits atherosclerosis in nonhuman primates. Hypertension 2005;46(5):1135–9.

[47] Schiffrin EL. Effects of aldosterone on the vasculature. Hypertension 2006;47(3):312–8.

[48] Yusuf S, Sleight P, Pogue J, et al. Effects of an angiotensin-converting-enzyme inhibitor, ramipril, on cardiovascular events in high-risk patients. The Heart Outcomes Prevention Evaluation Study Investigators. N Engl J Med 2000;342(3): 145–53.

Role of Neurohormonal Modulators in Heart Failure with Relatively Preserved Systolic Function

Jonathan A. Rapp, MD, Mihai Gheorghiade, MD*

Northwestern University Feinberg School of Medicine, Chicago, IL, USA

Cardiovascular disease remains the leading cause of mortality in the developed world and is responsible for nearly 1 million deaths per year in the United States [1]. Although the age-adjusted rates of death secondary to coronary artery disease (CAD) and stroke have decreased by approximately 50% in the last 10 years, there has been a large increase in the prevalence of heart failure (HF) [2,3].

It is estimated that 5 million Americans suffer from HF, and roughly 550,000 new cases are diagnosed annually [1]. HF was responsible for nearly 1 million hospital admissions in 2001 and is the most common discharge diagnosis in patients over 65 years of age. Furthermore, it is the primary cause of readmission within 60 days of discharge [1,4]. Approximately 330,000 patients die each year from HF, and the 1-year mortality rate of newly diagnosed patients approximates 20%. The total direct and indirect cost of managing this disease is expected to exceed $25 billion for 2004 [1].

Several echocardiographic cross-sectional studies have found that 40% to 71% of patients who have HF have relatively preserved systolic functions, a condition referred to as *diastolic heart failure* (DHF) [5–15]. In the last 15 years, several hospital-based studies have found that approximately 40% of patients admitted with worsening HF had DHF [16,17]. The most recently published database of patients who have HF found that approximately 40% of patients had an ejection fraction (EF) greater than 0.40 [18]. Although there are abundant data to guide the treatment of HF and systolic dysfunction (systolic heart failure, or SHF), evidence-based data are lacking in the management of DHF. This article examines the role of neurohormonal modulators in the management of DHF.

Definition and diagnosis

Definition

HF is a clinical syndrome that results from any functional or structural cardiac disorder that impairs the ability of the ventricles to fill with or eject blood. Symptoms include fatigue, poor exercise tolerance, dyspnea (exertional or resting), and signs and radiographic evidence of pulmonary and systemic congestion [19]. Standardized criteria for the diagnosis of HF have been described, such as those from the Framingham study [20]. Other tools, such as echocardiography and measurement of B-natriuretic peptide (BNP), also are used for diagnosis. BNP is a neurohormone secreted by the ventricles in response to muscle stretch caused by volume or pressure overload. Although it is a valuable marker of HF, it cannot be used to distinguish SHF from DHF [21,22] because patients often have components of both [23]. DHF is caused by diastolic dysfunction or, more specifically, abnormalities in active relaxation or passive stiffness of the left ventricle that result in abnormal left ventricular (LV) filling and elevated filling pressures [24,25].

This article originally appeared in *Heart Failure Clinics*, volume 1, issue 1.

* Corresponding author. Feinberg Cardiovascular Research Institute, Northwestern University Feinberg School of Medicine, Galter 10-240, 201 East Huron Street, Chicago, IL 60611.

E-mail address: m-gheorghiade@northwestern.edu (M. Gheorghiade)

Diagnosis

The Working Group of the European Society of Cardiology first published diagnostic criteria for DHF in 1998. It suggested that DHF could be diagnosed if (1) the patient had HF symptoms, (2) there was evidence of a normal left ventricular ejection fraction (LVEF), and (3) there was evidence of abnormal LV diastolic stiffness, relaxation, or filling [26]. Vasan and Levy [27] modified these criteria and proposed categorizing DHF diagnosis as definite, probable, and possible. All patients were required to have signs and symptoms of HF as well as an LVEF greater than 0.50. Diagnosis of definite and probable DHF required LVEF to be measured within 72 hours of the HF event. Furthermore, diagnosis of definite DHF required evidence of diastolic dysfunction measured by catheterization.

Gandhi and colleagues [28] found that, among patients hospitalized for acute pulmonary edema, there was no significant difference in LVEF between the time of presentation and 72 hours later after compensation was achieved. This proved to be true in the presence of SHF and DHF and indicated that a measurement of systolic function during an acute setting may not be necessary to establish the diagnosis of DHF. Moreover, a study by Smith and colleagues [17] demonstrated that outcomes were similar in patients who had DHF whose LVEFs were examined on index admission or 6 to 12 months previously. Therefore, as long as no intervening event had occurred, DHF can be diagnosed using an LVEF greater than 0.50 within 6 to 12 months before the initial presentation of HF [17,25]. Piccini and colleagues [21] also stated that DHF can be diagnosed without a measurement of diastolic function if the patient has (1) HF symptoms, (2) LVEF greater than 0.50, and (3) no significant valvular or pericardial disease. Clinically, SHF and DHF often coexist, and their managements are similar.

A comparison of the clinical characteristics of patients who have diastolic heart failure and systolic heart failure

Patients who have DHF and SHF have differing clinical characteristics. In a recent hospital-based study examining the differences between patients who have HF, 55% of women with HF had relatively preserved systolic functions compared with 29% of men. Patients who had DHF also tended to be older than their counterparts with

SHF (71 years versus 67 years of age) [29]. The Acute Decompensated Heart Failure National Registry (ADHERE), the largest HF registry, also found that patients who had DHF were older (74.2 versus 69.9 years of age) and more likely to be women (62% versus 39%) than patients who had SHF [18]. These data are consistent with prior studies that showed that women comprise 70% to 75% of patients who have DHF, and such patients have a mean age of 70 to 75 years [30–32].

Patients who have SHF and DHF also differ in their associated comorbidities. The ADHERE registry documented that a higher percentage of patients who have DHF are diabetic (46% versus 42%) and have atrial fibrillation (AF) (21% versus 17%) when compared with patients who have SHF, but CAD was more frequent in patients who have SHF (61% versus 47%) [18].

Lenzen and colleagues [29] found generally similar results (Table 1). Patients who had DHF had a higher prevalence of AF (25% versus 23%), hypertension (59% versus 50%), renal insufficiency (69% versus 59%), and history of stroke (28% versus 26%) than patients who had SHF. Although diabetes mellitus and ischemic heart disease were prevalent in both populations, they were more so in patients who had SHF.

Treatment differences, which have been studied, are quite striking. Patients who have DHF are less likely to receive angiotensin-converting enzyme (ACE) inhibitors, angiotensin II receptor–blockers (ARBs), β-blockers, digoxin, or diuretics than are patients who have SHF. They are, however, more likely to receive calcium-channel blockers [29–32].

Prognosis

Unfortunately, prognosis is poor for patients who have either SHF or DHF. Among hospitalized patients, mortality is similar between the two groups. It is almost certain that any difference favoring DHF becomes insignificant 3 to 6 months after hospital discharge [17,33–35]. Community-based studies showed similar mortality rates between the two groups in patients more than 65 years of age. In patients less than 65 years of age, however, DHF carries a lower 1-year mortality rate than SHF (7%–9% versus 12%–19%, respectively) [36–40].

Mortality seems to be related to age and the degree of accompanying CAD. The DIG trial found that the 3-year mortality for DHF was as low as 9% in patients less than 50 years of age but

Table 1
Comorbidities of patients with heart failure and with or without systolic dysfunction

| | Patients with known left ventricular function | | | |
Characteristic	PLVF n = 31,348	LVSD n = 3658	P value[a]	Patients not in this analysis n = 3895
Age (mean, SD)	71 Â ± 12 y	67 Â ± 13 y	<.001	76 Â ± 11.6 y
Women	1739 (55%)	1065 (29%)	<.001	2216 (57%)
Men > 70 y	666 (21%)	961 (26%)	<.001	1039 (27%)
Women > 70 y	1099 (35%)	607 (17%)	<.001	1748 (45%)
Comorbidity				
Hypertension	1845 (59%)	1829 (50%)	<.001	2005 (52%)
Diabetes mellitus	816 (26%)	1016 (28%)	.09	1075 (28%)
Ischemic heart disease	1851 (59%)	2508 (69%)	<.001	2060 (53%)
Previous revascularization	377 (12%)	674 (18%)	<.001	291 (8%)
Renal insufficiency	155 (5%)	220 (6%)	.05	296 (8%)
Prior stroke	492 (16%)	501 (14%)	.02	814 (21%)
Chronic atrial fibrillation	795 (25%)	827 (23%)	.01	860 (22%)
LVEF (mean, SD)	56 Â ± 9.8%	33 Â ± 10.9%	<.001	NA
Specialty at admission				
General internal medicine	1299 (42%)	1164 (32%)	<.001	2659 (68%)
Cardiology/cardiovascular surgery	1615 (51%)	2288 (63%)	<.001	769 (20%)
Duration of index hospitalization (median, IQR)	10 d (6–16)	10 d (6–15)	.26	9 d (5–14)
Contribution of heart failure to index admission	1189 (38%)	1904 (52%)	<.001	1141 (29%)

Abbreviations: IQR, interquartile range; LVEF, left ventricular ejection fraction; LVSD, left ventricular systolic dysfunction; NA, not available; PLVF, preserved left ventricular function; SD, standard deviation.

[a] Statistical difference between PLVF and LVSD

From Lenzen MJ, Scholte op Reimer WJM, Boersma E, et al. Differences between patients with a preserved and a depressed left ventricular function: a report from the EuroHeart Failure Survey. Eur Heart J 2004;25:1214–20; with permission.

as high as 39% in patients more than 80 years of age [41]. The Coronary Artery Surgery Study (CASS) found that the number of diseased vessels in patients who have DHF correlated with 3-year mortality (8% with no disease, 17% in one- or two-vessel disease, and 32% with triple-vessel disease) [42]. Results of morbidity studies mirror those of mortality studies. In community-based studies, the hospitalization rate for HF or a cardiovascular cause is lower in patients who have DHF than in those who have SHF [38,40]. Among hospitalized patients, the all-cause or HF readmission rates are similar in patients less than 80 years of age, regardless of type of HF (the all-cause readmission rate is approximately 45% at 6 months) [17,34,35]. In patients over 80 years of age, readmission rates for those who have SHF are higher than for those who have DHF [17].

Pathophysiology

The pathophysiology of DHF is understood best by dividing the disease into (1) intrinsic

processes that describe the pathologic changes in the myocardium itself and include mechanical, molecular, and neurohormonal factors, and (2) extrinsic processes that consist of the morbidities that cause the intrinsic changes. These morbidities include age, hypertension, CAD, AF, and diabetes mellitus (Fig. 1). Understanding the intrinsic processes is important because research into them may provide novel approaches to future therapy. The importance of the extrinsic factors cannot be overstated, however, because they create and worsen DHF and serve as the primary targets of current medical therapy. DHF also can be caused by infiltrative or restrictive cardiomyopathies (eg, amyloidosis, sarcoidosis, and hemochromatosis), but this article does not discuss these conditions [43].

Intrinsic processes

Ventricular relaxation

During systole, the left ventricle contracts and twists on its own axis. While blood is ejected, potential energy is stored in the ventricular

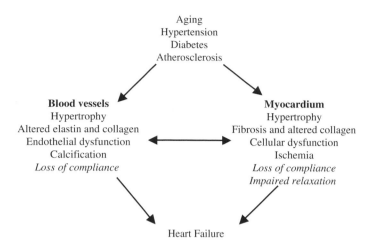

Fig. 1. Extrinsic diseases that bring about diastolic heart failure. Hypertension, coronary artery disease, atrial fibrillation, and diabetes mellitus serve as the primary targets of therapy for diastolic heart failure. (*From* Massie BM. Natriuretic peptide measurements for the diagnosis of "nonsystolic" heart failure: good news and bad. J Am Coll Cardiol 2003;41:2018–21; with permission.)

myofibrils that creates the torsion forces necessary for the ensuing ventricular suction and diastolic filling [44,45]. Echocardiographic studies have demonstrated that the extent of ventricular systolic twist highly correlates with mitral inflow acceleration and early diastolic filling [46]. Oblique fiber shortening is the most significant factor contributing to systolic twist and consequent filling [47]. During isovolumic relaxation, the left ventricle untwists about its axis without any blood movement between the cardiac chambers. This creates an intraventricular pressure gradient whose suction effect assists blood entry from the atrium into the ventricle once the mitral valve opens [48]. This process is normally responsible for roughly 70% of transmitral flow. β-Adrenergic stimulation may enhance the suction effect by increasing the rate and degree of ventricular pressure decline [49]. This effect is most critical during exercise, when it allows for increased diastolic filling volume without increased filling pressures. This effect is obtained while shortening the diastolic filling time [43].

Intracellular calcium handling seems to play a major role in ventricular relaxation. For contracted myocytes to relax and return to their resting length, actin-myosin bonds must be lysed through ATP-mediated processes in which calcium first dissociates from troponin-c and is then sequestered into the sarcoplasmic reticulum. This latter process is performed by the sarcoplasmic reticulum-calcium ATPase (SERCA) pump. The rate and degree of these cellular processes dictate the rate and degree of ventricular active relaxation [50]. Decreases in either the levels or activity of SERCA or increased levels of the SERCA inhibitor protein phospholamban can increase the amount of cytosolic calcium, thereby inhibiting the molecular processes required for myocyte relaxation and lengthening. Such events can occur in myocardial ischemia [51–53] or hypertrophy [54,55], two common circumstances in which diastolic dysfunction and failure occur.

Heart rate influences intracellular calcium concentration and transport [21]. In a patient who has defective calcium metabolism, increased heart rate can result in the accumulation of intracellular calcium ions and eventual calcium overload. This may yield prolonged interaction between actin and myosin, thus resulting in a state of prolonged myocardial contraction and possible impairment of diastolic function [56]. Additionally, tachycardia per se may hinder diastolic filling as a simple function of time: a faster heart rate results in less time for blood to enter the ventricles.

Ventricular compliance

Ventricular compliance is a function of mass and myocardial composition. Intracellular and extracellular structures influence compliance [50]. Titin is an intracellular protein component of the myocyte cytoskeleton. It is compressed during systole, and potential energy is stored. It returns to its resting length during diastole, like a spring, and contributes to the heart's diastolic relaxation. The degree of relaxation of titin is limited, thus protecting the sarcomere from excessive stretching. A change in titin isoform decreases compliance [57,58].

Alterations in collagen, an extracellular protein, also can impair diastolic function through its effects on ventricular compliance. Changes in the amount, distribution, type, degree of cross-linking, or geometry can be implicated [59–61]. Collagen synthesis can be altered by many physiologic circumstances, including neurohormonal activation, changes in preload or afterload, and changes in growth factor concentrations [21].

Neurohormonal factors in diastolic heart failure

In addition to the systemic renin–angiotensin–aldosterone system (RAAS), growing evidence supports the existence of a RAAS within the heart that may contribute to diastolic dysfunction [62–64]. Several observations have been made in hypertrophied hearts regarding the RAAS. For example, an infusion of angiotensin I in rats immediately impaired diastolic relaxation in hypertrophied, but not nonhypertrophied, hearts [64]. The hypertrophied hearts also had a greater ability to convert angiotensin I to angiotensin II [64]. Furthermore, after exposure to angiotensin II, hypertrophied hearts showed an exaggerated diastolic dysfunction during low-flow ischemia and a greater degree of ischemic diastolic dysfunction compared with nonhypertrophied hearts [65]. ACE inhibitors reduce the ischemia-mediated exaggeration of diastolic dysfunction in hypertrophied, but not in nonhypertrophied, hearts [65]. Angiotensin II, however, increases ischemic diastolic dysfunction even in nonhypertrophied hearts [66].

Aldosterone has deleterious effects on cardiac remodeling, specifically those that cause myocardial fibrosis. Cardiomyocytes, endothelial cells, and fibroblasts of the human heart all contain mineralocorticoid receptors that can be activated by aldosterone [67]. Such activation results in several events that increase myocardial fibrosis. There is up-regulation of the Na+/K+ ATPase in the heart that promotes events to induce fibroblast growth and collagen synthesis [68,69]. Aldosterone stimulates translation of the genes for types I and III collagen and fibrillar collagen [70]. It also alters coronary vascular permeability that may result in the exposure of fibroblasts to growth factors such as platelet-derived growth factor, which would increase collagen synthesis further [71,72]. Fibrosis begins as an accumulation of fibrillar collagen within the adventitia of the intramuscular coronary arteries, but eventually extends into the intracellular spaces [59,71]. Ultimately, aldosterone causes interstitial and perivascular myocardial fibrosis.

Extrinsic processes

Age

As noted, age is a major risk factor for DHF. Aging is associated with an increase in myocardial collagen, decreased β-receptor responsiveness [73], and impaired calcium ion handling because of decreased levels of SERCA [74], all of which lead to abnormal relaxation or altered myocardial elasticity. Aortic stiffness also increases with age, increasing afterload and causing LV hypertrophy, which may add to ventricular stiffness [75].

Hypertension

Hypertension is the most common risk factor for the development of DHF [21]. Hypertension has been associated with irregular myocardial high-energy phosphate metabolism [76] that may lower cytosolic concentrations of ATP [77]. This may cause malfunction of the SERCA, calcium overload, and impaired diastolic relaxation [43,78]. Hypertension also creates a high LV afterload that can retard relaxation and cause elevated filling pressures and a decreased end-diastolic volume [79]. This leads to increased ventricular wall tension that induces myocardial stretching and activation of neurohormonal systems, such as those that increase production of angiotensin II [80]. These events trigger altered gene expression with subsequent cell growth and extracellular matrix changes that further contribute to increased LV mass and stiffness [81].

Coronary artery disease

CAD can induce diastolic dysfunction in two major ways. First, infarcted muscle can result in scarring, fibrosis, and compensatory hypertrophy of healthy myocardium, all of which yield non-compliant tissue. Second, ischemia can cause calcium ion sequestration into the sarcoplasmic reticulum during ATP-dependent relaxation [43,51]. Notably, when diastolic dysfunction is present in the early phases of an acute myocardial infarction (MI), there is an increased association between the development of in-hospital HF and cardiac death within 1 year [82].

Atrial fibrillation

AF is of special concern in patients who have DHF. Atrial contraction is usually responsible for less than 30% of the forward flow from the atrium to the ventricle but can become critically important when LV filling pressures are high secondary to diastolic dysfunction. Loss of coordinated atrial contraction can lead to decreased ventricular filling, particularly when associated with a rapid ventricular response, and may lead rapidly to pulmonary congestion [83].

Diabetes mellitus

Diabetes mellitus is associated with diastolic dysfunction and HF. Several studies have identified diabetes mellitus as a major risk factor for the development of HF, including the Studies of Left Ventricular Dysfunction (SOLVD), the Heart Outcomes Prevention Evaluation (HOPE) trial, and the Cardiovascular Health Study [84–86]. Recent work examining the relationship between diabetes mellitus and DHF has found that diastolic dysfunction may be the first stage of diabetic cardiomyopathy [87,88]. Zalbalgoitia and colleagues [89] found that over 40% of patients who had diabetes mellitus had some form of diastolic dysfunction, and abnormal LV relaxation seems to correlate with hemoglobin A_{1C} levels [90,91]. Similar findings were confirmed in the Strong Heart Study, which found that Native Americans who had diabetes mellitus tended to have higher rates of echocardiographic evidence of diastolic dysfunction independent of age, systolic function, blood pressure, or LV mass [90].

The pathologic changes seen in the diabetic heart consist of increased matrix collagen, myocyte hypertrophy, intramyocardial microangiopathy, and interstitial fibrosis [92]. These morphologic abnormalities likely result from altered myocardial glucose and fatty acid metabolism associated with diabetes mellitus [21]. Diabetes mellitus causes advanced glycosylated end products (AGEs) that affect several aspects of cardiac microanatomy and physiology. Once AGEs develop in the arterial walls and myocardial tissue, they form cross-links to local collagen fibers, thereby decreasing distensbility of the blood vessels and myocardium [93]. Furthermore, AGEs and reactive oxygen species can affect calcium handling, ion channels, mitochondrial function, and apoptosis; these processes lead to diastolic and systolic dysfunction [93]. Additional changes noted in patients who have diabetes mellitus include impaired β-receptor signal transduction and induction of the fetal gene pattern [94,95]. This gene pattern favors expression of an isoform of the Î±-myosin heavy chain (β-myosin heavy chain) that has slower ATPase activity than its adult isoform [96]. There is also down-regulation of the SERCA gene resulting in abnormal calcium homeostasis [97,98]. This further contributes to diastolic dysfunction [99].

Treatment

With the exception of the Candesartan in Heart Failure: Assessment of Reduction in Mortality and Morbidity (CHARM)-Preserved [100] and Digitalis Investigation Group (DIG) studies [41], no large, randomized, double-blind, placebo-controlled trial results are available to direct the management of patients who have DHF. Therefore, treatment is based largely on results from smaller clinical studies, personal experience, and, most important, the control of the extrinsic processes known to create and exacerbate DHF (ie, hypertension, CAD, AF/tachycardia, and diabetes mellitus) [50]. Fortunately, there is a wealth of clinical data to guide the latter therapy, much of which focuses on neurohormonal modulation. After briefly discussing symptom control, this article reviews the evidence-based literature in the treatment of DHF and then focuses on the role of neurohormonal modulators in the management of the conditions that contribute to DHF.

Symptom control

The initial goal in the treatment of DHF is symptomatic relief, which is achieved by decreasing pulmonary congestion. Therapeutic goals may include diastolic volume reduction (with the objective of lowering LV diastolic pressure), maintenance of sinus rhythm, or increasing the duration of diastole by slowing the ventricular rate [50].

Diastolic volume and, thereby, LV diastolic filling pressure can be lowered in several ways. First, total body volume can be reduced with the use of diuretics and fluid or sodium restriction. Second, preload can be reduced with the use of nitrates. Third, blockade of the RAAS by ACE inhibitors, ARBs, or aldosterone antagonists may be employed [50].

Because of the dependence on atrial contraction for ventricular filling in patients who have DHF, AF must be treated aggressively. Optimally, sinus rhythm can be maintained, but if this is not possible, rate control is a necessity [19]. Preventing tachycardia is important for symptom control because it may lead to incomplete ventricular relaxation, pulmonary congestion, and, therefore, symptoms [50]. Blood pressure should be kept below 130/80 in accordance with current American College of Cardiology/American Heart Association guidelines [19]. All patients suspected of having an ischemic etiology of HF should be treated appropriately medically and investigated for revascularization [19]. Anti-ischemic medications such as nitrates, β-blockers, and calcium channel blockers should be used as necessary.

Evidence-based review of treatment for diastolic heart failure

DIG, the first large randomized study, evaluated the effects of digoxin on mortality (the primary endpoint) and cardiovascular death, death from worsening HF, HF hospitalization, and hospitalization for other causes (the secondary endpoints) in patients who had HF [41]. The study was conducted over 3 to 5 years in patients who had HF and normal sinus rhythm. There were two trials: the main trial included patients with LVEF of 0.45 or less, and the ancillary trial studied patients with LVEF greater than 0.45. This discussion focuses on the ancillary trial.

Patients were assigned to receive digoxin (n = 492) or placebo (n = 496). Dosing was calculated by an algorithm according to the patient's age, sex, weight, and renal function. The two groups shared similar baseline characteristics. Examples of recorded statistics were age, sex, LVEF, New York Heart Association (NYHA) class, number of signs or symptoms of HF, dose of study medication, and concomitant medications (diuretics, ACE inhibitors, nitrates, or other vasodilators). There were 115 deaths (23.4%) in the digoxin group and 116 deaths (23.4%) in the placebo group, yielding a risk ratio of 0.99. With respect to the combined outcome of death and hospitalization from worsening HF, the risk ratio was 0.82 in favor of the digoxin group; most of the benefit was seen in rates of hospitalization. The results of this study indicate that digoxin provides a benefit in HF morbidity but not in mortality.

The CHARM-Preserved trial [100] studied the effects of an angiotensin-receptor blocker, candesartan, on the composite outcome of cardiovascular mortality or hospital admission caused by worsening HF. Several secondary outcomes were assessed, including nonfatal MI, nonfatal stroke,

and coronary revascularization. Three thousand twenty-three patients were randomized to either candesartan therapy or placebo. Mean follow-up was 36.6 months. LVEF was required to be greater than 0.40. The mean age was 67 years, and approximately 26% of patients were 75 or more years of age. The mean LVEF was 54%. Approximately 60% of patients were NYHA class II. Roughly 56% of patients had an ischemic cause of their HF, and over 28% had coexisting diabetes mellitus. Most patients were treated with β-blockers, diuretics, and antiplatelet agents, whereas less than half received ACE inhibitors, spironolactone, calcium channel blockers, digoxin, or lipid-lowering agents. The target dose of study drug was 32 mg/d.

The primary outcome occurred in 22% of patients in the candesartan group compared with 24% of patients in the placebo group (Fig. 2). Most of the benefit was from a 29% reduction in the number of congestive heart failure (CHF) hospitalizations in the candesartan group. The cardiovascular mortality was 11% in both groups. The low mortality likely was related to patient selection, with most patients having NYHA class II HF. Ultimately, the investigators described a trend in favor of using candesartan for the prevention of cardiovascular outcomes in their study population, but the difference in the primary outcome was modest and of borderline significance.

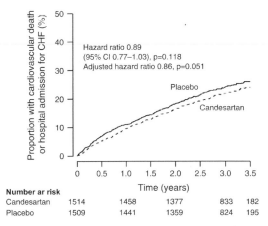

Fig. 2. Results of the CHARM-Preserved trial. There was no statistically significant benefit in primary outcome in the study: cardiovascular death or hospital admission for congestive heart failure. (*From* Yusuf S, Pfeffer MA, Swedberg K, et al. Effects of candesartan in patients with chronic HF and preserved left-ventricular ejection fraction: the CHARM-Preserved Trial. Lancet 2003;362:777–81; with permission.)

Secondary outcomes did not reach statistical significance. There was a 40% reduction in the diagnosis of new-onset diabetes mellitus in the candesartan group. This finding has implications for the future treatment of DHF and longer-term follow-up is perhaps necessary. Notably, DIG [41] and CHARM-Preserved [100] demonstrated that much of the morbidity and mortality associated with DHF patients was unrelated to DHF per se, a fact thay may have contributed to the negative results in these trials.

Neurohormonal modulation in the treatment of conditions that contribute to diastolic heart failure

ACE-inhibitors, ARBs, β-blockers, and aldosterone antagonists are neurohormonal modulators that influence hypertension, CAD, atrial fibrillation, diabetes mellitus, or have direct effects on myocardium. These medications form the backbone of treatment for DHF because they are effective in the treatment of the underlying cardiovascular diseases that can lead or contribute to DHF.

Angiotensin-converting enzyme inhibitors
Hypertension. ACE inhibitors are considered the cornerstone of therapy in many patients who have cardiovascular disease. The antihypertensive effect of ACE inhibitors is accepted widely, which is of primary importance in their role in the treatment of DHF. Although studies such as the Antihypertensive and Lipid-Lowering Treatment to Prevent Heart Attack Trial [101] and those discussed below document blood pressure reduction with use of these agents, this article focuses on trials that have demonstrated other beneficial effects of ACE inhibitors on the conditions that contribute to DHF.

Coronary artery disease. HOPE is one of many studies showing the benefits of ACE inhibitors [102]. In this study, over 9200 patients at high risk for cardiovascular events were assigned to receive either ramipril, 10 mg/d orally, or placebo to assess the effects of ramipril on cardiovascular outcomes. Patients were followed for up to 5 years and were 55 or more years of age with a history of CAD, stroke, peripheral vascular disease, or diabetes mellitus plus at least one other cardiovascular risk factor (hypertension, elevated cholesterol levels, low high-density lipoprotein levels, cigarette smoking, or documented microalbuminuria).

The investigators found a statistically significant reduction in the ramipril group compared

with the placebo group for the primary endpoint of MI, stroke, or death caused by cardiovascular causes (14% versus 17.8%) as well as death from cardiovascular causes (6.1% versus 8.1%), MI (9.9% versus 12.3%), stroke (3.4% versus 4.9%), and all-cause mortality (10.4% versus 12.2%). The need for revascularization also was decreased in the ramipril group (16% versus 18.3%). HF occurred in 9% of the ramipril group and 11.5% of the placebo group. The investigators noted that the results were independent of blood pressure–lowering effects alone because most patients did not have hypertension at baseline and the mean blood pressure reduction was only 3/2 mm Hg. They speculated that the benefits of ACE inhibition may result from blocking angiotensin II–mediated vasoconstriction [103], inhibiting vascular smooth muscle cell proliferation [103], preventing plaque rupture [104], or reducing LV hypertrophy [102,103].

More recently, the European Trial on Reduction of Cardiac Events with Perindopril in Stable Coronary Artery Disease (EUROPA) investigated a similar question with a different ACE inhibitor [105]. This trial included patients 18 or more years of age without evidence of HF and with a history of stable CAD—defined as a history of MI (64%), percutaneous or surgical coronary revascularization (55%), or angiographic evidence of at least 70% stenosis of at least one major coronary artery (61%). Men were included if they had a positive stress test (5%). The investigators compared the ability of perindopril, 8 mg/d orally, with placebo in preventing death, MI, or cardiac arrest in patients without HF or excessive hypertension. The mean follow-up was 4.2 years. Cardiovascular mortality, MI, or cardiac arrest was reduced in the perindopril group (8.0% versus 9.9%). The reduction in frequency of clinical MI and cardiovascular death was similar to that found in HOPE (20% versus 21%, respectively). Both trials allowed concomitant treatment with medications such as β-blockers, diuretics, aspirin, and others.

Atrial fibrillation. A substudy of the Trandolapril Cardiac Evaluation (TRACE) was the first to suggest that ACE inhibitors prevent AF in some patients [106]. Patients were assigned to receive either trandolapril or placebo on day 3 to 7 after an acute MI. Trandolapril was titrated up to 4 mg/d as tolerated, and patients were followed for 2 to 4 years. The patients had normal sinus rhythm at baseline, were over 18 years of age, were admitted to the hospital for an acute MI, and displayed impaired LV dysfunction by echocardiography (LVEF < 0.36). The investigators found that placebo-treated patients were more than twice as likely to develop AF than trandolapril-treated patients (5.3% versus 2.3%).

Vermes and colleagues [107] reported a similar finding in their retrospective analysis of patients from the Montreal Heart Institute included in the SOLVD trial. Patients who had AF on a baseline electrocardiogram were excluded. The average length of follow-up was 3 years. Of the 55 patients who developed AF, there was a statistically significant difference: 10 (5.4%) were in the enalapril group and 45 (24%) were in the placebo group.

Diabetes mellitus. ACE inhibitors also have an effect on the development of diabetes mellitus. The HOPE trial demonstrated a statistically significant reduction in new-onset diabetes mellitus in those taking ramipril (3.6% versus 5.4%) [102]. Although there was no comment on the reduction of diabetes mellitus in the EUROPA trial, the CAPPP study demonstrated that captopril, like ramipril, was associated with a statistically significant reduction in the diagnosis of new-onset diabetes mellitus [108].

Direct effects on myocardium. Several studies have documented a reduction in myocardial mass with ACE inhibitor therapy, such as the 4E study discussed below [109]. More recently, however, Brilla and colleagues [110] described the lisinopril-mediated regression of myocardial fibrosis in patients who have hypertensive heart disease. This study examined 35 patients who had primary hypertension, left ventricular hypertrophy (LVH), and LV diastolic dysfunction. Patients were randomized to receive either lisinopril or hydrochlorothiazide (HCTZ). Left heart catheterization with endomyocardial biopsy, Doppler echocardiography, and 24-hour blood pressure monitoring were performed at baseline and at 6 months. The primary endpoint was myocardial fibrosis (directly measured by the collagen volume fraction and myocardial hydroxyproline concentration), and the secondary endpoints were blood pressure, LVH as determined by LV mass index and myocyte diameter, and LV diastolic function assessed using parameters to measure relaxation and myocardial stiffness.

In the lisinopril group, the collagen volume fraction was reduced from a mean of 6.9% to

a mean of 6.3% and the myocardial hydroxyproline concentration decreased from an average of 9.9 μg/mg to 8.3 μg/mg of LV weight ($P < .05$ and $P < .00001$ compared with the HCTZ group, respectively). This was associated with an increase in the ratio of early to late diastolic filling (E:A ratio) from a mean of 0.72 to a mean of 0.91 ($P < .05$ versus HCTZ) and a decrease in isovolumic relaxation time from a mean of 123 milliseconds to a mean of 81 milliseconds ($P < .00002$ versus HCTZ). The A-wave duration of transmitral flow during atrial contraction was improved significantly in the lisinopril group compared with the HCTZ group ($P < .0002$), indicating that there was a reduction in ventricular stiffness in the lisinopril group, but there was no statistically significant change in either group when the stiffness constant k was assessed. Normalized blood pressure did not alter the results significantly. No regression in LVH occurred in the lisinopril-treated patients, whereas the HCTZ group experienced a decrease in myocyte diameter from a mean of 22.1 μm to a mean of 20.7 μm ($P < .01$ compared with lisinopril). The important finding is that lisinopril altered myocardial fibrosis and concomitantly improved diastolic function [110].

Clearly, ACE inhibitors play a significant role in the treatment and prevention of entities that contribute to DHF, specifically hypertension, CAD, AF, diabetes mellitus, and unhealthy ventricular remodeling and myocardial fibrosis.

Angiotensin II–receptor blockers
Hypertension. Like ACE inhibitors, ARBs modify several of the disease processes that contribute to DHF. Their power to reduce hypertension has been documented in several trials [111–113], and the current discussion will focus on trials that demonstrate other beneficial effects.

Coronary artery disease. The Valsartan Antihypertensive Long-Term Use Evaluation (VALUE) tested the hypothesis that, despite similar blood pressure reduction, valsartan would reduce cardiac morbidity and mortality more effectively than amlodipine [111]. Patients were 50 or more years of age, had treated or untreated baseline hypertension, and had a combination of predefined risk factors, including diabetes mellitus, smoking, proteinuria by urine dipstick, and elevated total cholesterol. Patients were followed for 4 to 6 years. The primary outcome of time to first major cardiac event and the development of HF were not significantly different between the two groups. The valsartan group did, however, demonstrate a statistically significant difference in the rate of MI compared with the amlodipine group, 4.1% versus 4.8%, respectively. Blood pressure was reduced by both medications, although more so for amlodipine.

The Losartan Intervention for Endpoint Reduction in Hypertension (LIFE) study investigated if blocking the angiotensin-II receptor with losartan would improve LVH beyond blood pressure reduction and, subsequently, lower cardiovascular morbidity and mortality [112]. The investigators included patients 55 to 80 years of age who had previously treated or untreated hypertension and LVH, as determined by electrocardiogram. Patients who had an MI or stroke within the last 6 months, angina requiring treatment with β-blockers or calcium channel blockers, CHF, or LVEF less than 0.40 were excluded. Mean follow-up was 4.8 years.

The study found that a composite endpoint of stroke, MI, or cardiovascular death was decreased in the losartan patients compared with those who were assigned atenolol for a similar blood pressure reduction (23.8% versus 27.9%, respectively). Additionally, a new diagnosis of diabetes mellitus was made more frequently in the atenolol group compared with the losartan group (17.4% versus 13%, respectively). There was no statistically significant difference in admission for HF. Importantly, blood pressure was reduced similarly in the losartan and atenolol groups (reductions of 30.2/16.6 and 29.1/16.8, respectively); therefore it is likely that the beneficial effects of the ARB extended beyond blood pressure control.

Atrial fibrillation. Like ACE inhibitors, ARBs may help prevent AF. Madrid and colleagues [114] investigated irbesartan in maintaining sinus rhythm following conversion from AF. Patients were 18 or more years of age, had AF for more than 7 days, and were randomized to either amiodarone, 400 mg/d orally, or amiodarone plus irbesartan, 150 to 300 mg/d orally. There were several exclusion criteria, including cardiac surgery within 3 months, MI during the previous 6 months, unstable angina, and NYHA class IV HF. Medical therapy was started after anticoagulation to an international normalized ratio above 2.0 and electrical cardioversion was scheduled for 3 weeks later. At 2-month follow-up, 84.79% of the amiodarone group had AF compared with only 63.16% of the

dual therapy group. Results were statistically significant.

Diabetes mellitus. Similar to ACE inhibitors, ARBs may be beneficial in the prevention of diabetes mellitus. The VALUE trial found that new-onset diabetes mellitus was far less frequent in the valsartan group than the amlodipine group (32.1% versus 41.1%) [111].

Direct effects on myocardium. The LIFE study demonstrated a final benefit of ARBs. Losartan-based therapy reduced LVH (and to a greater degree than the atenolol-based therapy) based on electrocardiogram criteria and echocardiographic studies [112,115]. The mean Cornell voltage-duration product was reduced by 290 and 124 mm/ms in the losartan and atenolol groups, respectively. The Sokolow-Lyon voltage was reduced by 4.6 and 2.7 mm, respectively [112]. Reduced hypertrophy may be yet another way in which ARBs can improve diastolic dysfunction. Thus, compared with ACE inhibitors, ARBs are acceptable alternatives for the treatment for DHF because of their effects on LVH and on the underlying conditions of DHF.

β-Blockers

Hypertension. A wealth of literature supports the use of selective and nonselective β-receptor antagonists in many conditions, making them one of the most important classes of medications in cardiology. The blood-pressure lowering effects of β-blockers have been well documented and are generally accepted [116–119]. These agents have been used to treat hypertension for over 30 years [119].

Coronary artery disease. β-Blockers also play a role in the treatment of CAD. In the Norwegian Multicenter Study Group trial, 1884 post-MI patients were assigned randomly to timolol, 5 mg/d orally starting dose, with a goal of 20 mg/d orally, or placebo [120]. Therapy was started 7 to 28 days after infarction, and patients were followed for 12 to 33 months. All-cause mortality was reduced by 39%, sudden death by 45%, and nonfatal reinfarction by 28% in the timolol group.

In the Beta-blocker Heart Attack Trial (BHAT), over 3800 patients were monitored following an acute MI [121,122]. Five to twenty-one days post-MI, patients were assigned randomly to receive either propranolol, 180 to 240 mg/d orally, or placebo. Patients were followed for an average of 24 months (the study was ended

9 months prematurely). The propranolol group showed a 26% reduction in all-cause mortality, a 28% reduction in sudden death, and a 23% reduction in all-cause mortality and reinfarction (all reductions were statistically significant). Although not statistically significant, the propranolol group had lower rates of reinfarction than the placebo group when this endpoint was measured independently (10% versus 13%).

Although the Norwegian and BHAT studies were done before the modern era of treatments for CAD such as ACE inhibitors, statins, or interventional techniques, their benefits in post-MI patients have been confirmed in other trials, such as the Survival and Ventricular Enlargement (SAVE) and Acute Infarction Ramipril Efficacy (AIRE) trials [123,124].

Atrial fibrillation. β-Blockers are useful in patients who have AF or other tachycardic states. Maintaining a resting heart rate between 60 and 70 beats per minute and blunting exercise-induced tachycardia may prevent LV pressure elevation and pulmonary congestion by mechanisms previously discussed, thereby providing symptomatic relief [21,50]. Recent studies have validated that rate control is an acceptable, if not preferable, goal of therapy in AF and that β-blockers are effective rate-controlling agents in AF [125,126]. Furthermore, after cardioversion, β-blockers are effective agents for maintaining sinus rhythm [127].

Direct effects on myocardium. As with the other medications in this article, β-blockers reduce LVH, although by a lesser degree than other antihypertensive medications [128]. In their meta-analysis of 50 studies, Schmieder and colleagues [128] found that β-blockers were associated with a 4.5% reduction in LV mass index. ACE inhibitors and diuretics, however, were associated with 11.8% and 8.6% reductions in LV mass index, respectively.

Three recent studies have demonstrated that carvedilol has a beneficial effect on diastolic function. In 27 patients who had LV systolic dysfunction, carvedilol therapy favorably modified diastolic filling, independent of systolic function. A restrictive filling pattern, related to an unfavorable prognosis, changed to pseudonormal or altered relaxation during treatment with carvedilol. The results of Doppler ultrasound after 4 months showed a significant increase of A wave, deceleration time, and isovolumic relaxation time.

These improvements were increased to a greater extent at 1 year and were not seen in the placebo group [129].

A study that treated 45 patients who had HF (LVEF = 0.24) with carvedilol showed that long-term therapy with this β-blocker prevented or partially reversed progressive LV dilatation. The effects on LV remodeling were associated with a concomitant significant recovery of diastolic reserve and a significant decrease of mitral regurgitation [130].

Finally, a study including 113 patients who had preserved systolic dysfunction and DHF showed that carvedilol significantly improved the E/A ratio versus placebo. Carvedilol improved diastolic filling compared with placebo, and patients with higher heart rates showed particular benefit [131]. Further investigation into the beneficial effects of β-blockers in DHF should be pursued.

Aldosterone-receptor antagonists

Hypertension. Aldosterone receptor-blockers, such as spironolactone and eplerenone, are potassium-sparing diuretics that have blood pressure–lowering effects in addition to other effects [132]. Eplerenone, which differs from spironolactone in that it has reduced progesterone and androgen-receptor effects, reduces blood pressure an average of 6/4 to 24/14 mm Hg, depending on the dose [132]. Comparative trials have shown that eplerenone has similar antihypertensive effects to those of enalapril, amlodipine, losartan, and spironolactone [132–135].

Direct effects on myocardium. Spironolactone reduces the density of angiotensin-I receptors brought about by aldosterone, suppresses vascular angiotensin-II conversion, improves endothelial function hindered by aldosterone, and inhibits aldosterone-induced interstitial and perivascular fibrosis [136–140]. Spironolactone also can prevent cardiac and arterial fibrosis, improving the overall hemodynamic circumstances that create diastolic dysfunction [141]. Chronic treatment with spironolactone reduces LV mass and plasma markers of myocardial fibrosis [142,143].

Eplerenone has similar effects to those of spironolactone. It significantly reduces cardiac hypertrophy in experimental models [144] as well as improves ventricular remodeling in HF [145]. Studies such as the 4E-Left Ventricular Hypertrophy Study have confirmed eplerenone's beneficial effects in reducing LV mass in patients who have hypertension, similar to the effects seen with spironolactone [109]. In that study, patients who received eplerenone, 200 mg/d orally, were compared with those who received enalapril, 40 mg/d orally, and patients who received a combination of eplerone 200 mg/d orally and enalapril 10 mg/d orally. The primary endpoint was change from baseline LV mass at either 9 months or at the time of study discontinuation. LV mass was assessed using MRI. The investigators found that eplerenone resulted in an adjusted mean decrease of 14.5 g in LV mass compared with 19.7 g for enalapril and 27.2 g for the combination group. The changes in LV mass and hypertrophy have important implications for the treatment of diastolic dysfunction. Moreover, although ACE inhibitors and ARBs reduce blood aldosterone levels initially, there is a rebound effect in which aldosterone levels increase over time after the initiation of blockade of the angiotensin system [146]. Therefore, aldosterone-blocking agents may prove to be key players in the treatment of DHF.

Although the role of neurohormonal modulators in the treatment of DHF needs to be studied in dedicated randomized, placebo-controlled trials, these medications have been well studied in the treatment of conditions that contribute to DHF. These medications are therefore state-of-the-art therapy for the treatment of DHF and should be used whenever necessary. Several trials evaluating treatment options in patients who have DHF are underway. The Perindopril for Elderly People With Chronic Heart Failure study is studying the effect of the ACE inhibitor perindopril in patients who have DHF. Two trials are examining the effects of ARBs (irbesartan and losartan), and another study is comparing perindopril with irbesartan and placebo in patients who have DHF. Finally, one trial is investigating the role of an agent that may improve calcium uptake in the sarcoplasmic reticulum (MCC-135) in the treatment of DHF [21]. The management of this increasingly prevalent disease will be defined better when the results of these trials are published and new trials are developed.

Additional treatment options

Several primary [147,148] and secondary [149–151] prevention trials have shown that statins reduce CAD morbidity and mortality rates and increase overall survival in patients who have cardiovascular disease. Through their influence in decreasing the rate of MI and their beneficial effects on CAD, they contribute to the treatment of DHF.

Given the significance of diabetes mellitus in DHF, glycemic control should be managed tightly in diabetic patients. Iribarren and colleagues [152] found that glycemic control reduces the risk of HF in patients who have diabetes mellitus. Unfortunately, there are no data available describing which glucose-altering medications provide the best reduction in HF [21].

Summary

Approximately 40% to 50% of patients who have clinical HF have DHF. DHF carries a significant burden of morbidity and mortality as well as cost to society. The major conditions associated with it are advanced age, hypertension, CAD, AF, and diabetes mellitus. Currently, there is a paucity of evidence-based data guiding the treatment of HF with a relatively preserved systolic function although several studies are in progress. The data from the two large, randomized trials that are available indicate that a significant percentage of these patients' morbidity and mortality stems from causes other than heart failure. The challenge for future researchers is to develop trials that overcome the age-associated morbidities and mortality of these patient's thereby producing studies that may yield positive results, thus improving the way DHF is managed.

Neurohormonal modulators such as ACE inhibitors, ARBs, β-blockers, and aldosterone-receptor antagonists are important tools in the treatment of DHF because of their indispensable roles in treating the underlying conditions known to cause diastolic dysfunction. As clinical and basic science research mounts, clinicians will have better defined options to attack this prevalent problem and, it is hoped, will change the poor prognosis that faces these patients.

References

[1] American Heart Association. Heart disease and stroke statistics—2004 update. Dallas (TX): American Heart Association; 2003.

[2] American Heart Association. 2002 heart and stroke statistical update. Dallas (TX): American Heart Association; 2003.

[3] Miller LW, Missov ED. Epidemiology of heart failure. Cardiol Clin 2001;19:547–55.

[4] Haldeman GA, Croft JB, Giles WH, et al. Hospitalization of patients with heart failure: National

Hospital Discharge Survey, 1985 to 1995. Am Heart J 1999;137:352–60.

[5] Hogg K, Swedlberg K, McMurray J. Heart failure with preserved left ventricular systolic function: epidemiology, clinical characteristics, and prognosis. J Am Coll Cardiol 2004;43:317–27.

[6] Cortina A, Reguero J, Segovia E, et al. Prevalence of heart failure in Asturias (a region in the north of Spain). Am J Cardiol 2001;87:1417–9.

[7] Mosterd A, Hoes AW, de Bruyne MC, et al. Prevalence of heart failure and left ventricular dysfunction in the general population: the Rotterdam Study. Eur Heart J 1999;20:447–55.

[8] Nielsen OW, Hilden J, Larsen CT, et al. Cross-sectional study estimating prevalence of heart failure and left ventricular systolic dysfunction in community patients at risk. Heart 2001;86:172–8.

[9] Hedberg P, Lonnberg I, Jonason T, et al. Left ventricular systolic dysfunction in 75-year-old men and women; a population-based study. Eur Heart J 2001;22:676–83.

[10] Morgan S, Smith H, Simpson I, et al. Prevalence and clinical characteristics of left ventricular dysfunction among elderly patients in general practice setting: cross-sectional survey. BMJ 1999;318: 368–72.

[11] Kupari M, Lindroos M, Iivanainen AM, et al. Congestive heart failure in old age: prevalence, mechanisms and 4-year prognosis in the Helsinki Ageing Study. J Intern Med 1997;241:387–94.

[12] Ceia F, Fonseca C, Mota T, et al, and the EPICA Investigators. Prevalence of chronic heart failure in Southwestern Europe: the EPICA study. Eur J Heart Fail 2002;4:531–9.

[13] Kitzman DW, Gardin JM, Gottdiener JS, et al. Importance of heart failure with preserved systolic function in patients > or = 65 years of age. CHS Research Group. Cardiovascular Health Study. Am J Cardiol 2001;87:413–9.

[14] Devereux RB, Roman MJ, Liu JE, et al. Congestive heart failure despite normal left ventricular systolic function in a population-based sample: the Strong Heart Study. Am J Cardiol 2000;86:1090–6.

[15] Redfield MM, Jacobsen SJ, Burnett JC Jr, et al. Burden of systolic and diastolic ventricular dysfunction in the community: appreciating the scope of the heart failure epidemic. JAMA 2003;289: 194–202.

[16] Vasan RS, Benjamin EJ, Levy D. Prevalence, clinical features and prognosis of diastolic heart failure: an epidemiologic perspective. J Am Coll Cardiol 1995;26:1565–74.

[17] Smith GL, Masoudi FA, Vaccarino V, et al. Outcomes in heart failure patients with preserved ejection fraction: mortality, readmission, and functional decline. J Am Coll Cardiol 2003;41: 1510–8.

[18] Fonarow GC for the ADHERE Scientific Advisory Committee. The Acute Decompensated Heart Failure National Registry (ADHERE): opportunities to improve care of patients hospitalized with acute decompensated heart failure. Rev Cardiovasc Med 2003;4(Suppl 7):S21–30.

[19] Hunt SA, Baker DW, Chin MH, et al. ACC/AHA guidelines for the evaluation and management of chronic heart failure in the adult: executive summary. A report of the American College of Cardiology/American Heart Association Task Force on Practice Guidelines (Committee to revise the 1995 Guidelines for the Evaluation and Management of Heart Failure). J Am Coll Cardiol 2001;38: 2101–13.

[20] McKee PA, Castelli WP, McNamara PM, et al. The natural history of congestive heart failure: the Framingham study. N Engl J Med 1971;285: 1441–6.

[21] Piccini JP, Klein L, Gheorghiade M, et al. New insights into diastolic heart failure: role of diabetes mellitus. Am J Med 2004;116(5A):64S–75S.

[22] Maisel AS, McCord J, Nowak RM, et al. Bedside B-type natriuretic peptide in the emergency diagnosis of heart failure with reduced or preserved ejection fraction. Results from the Breathing not Properly Multinational Study. J Am Coll Cardiol 2003;41:2018–21.

[23] Zile MR, Brutsaert DL. New concepts in diastolic dysfunction and diastolic heart failure: part I: diagnosis, prognosis, and measurements of diastolic function. Circulation 2002;105:1387–93.

[24] Zile MR, Catalin FB, Gaasch WH. Diastolic heart failure—abnormalities in active relaxation and passive stiffness of the left ventricle. N Engl J Med 2004;350:1953–9.

[25] Zile MR. Heart failure with preserved ejection fraction: is this diastolic heart failure? J Am Coll Cardiol 2003;41:1519–22.

[26] European Study Group on Diastolic Heart Failure. How to diagnose diastolic heart failure. Eur Heart J 1998;19:990–1003.

[27] Vasan RS, Levy D. Defining diastolic heart failure: a call for standardized diagnostic criteria. Circulation 2000;101:2118–21.

[28] Gandhi SK, Powers JC, Nomeir AM, et al. The pathogenesis of acute pulmonary edema associated with hypertension. N Engl J Med 2001;344:17–22.

[29] Lenzen MJ, Scholte op Reimer WJM, Boersma E, et al. Differences between patients with a preserved and a depressed left ventricular function: a report from the EuroHeart Failure Survey. Eur Heart J 2004;25:1214–20.

[30] Kitzman DW, Little WC, Brubaker PH, et al. Pathophysiological characterization of isolated diastolic heart failure in comparison to systolic heart failure. JAMA 2002;288:2144–50.

[31] Chen HH, Lainchbury JG, Senni M, et al. Diastolic heart failure in the community: clinical profile, natural history, therapy, and impact of proposed diagnostic criteria. J Card Fail 2002;8:279–87.

[32] McDermott MM, Feinglass J, Sy J, et al. Hospitalized congestive heart failure patients with preserved versus abnormal left ventricular systolic function: clinical characteristics and drug therapy. Am J Med 1995;99:629–35.

[33] Philbin EF, Rocco TA, Lindenmuth NW, et al. Systolic versus diastolic heart failure in the community practice: clinical features, outcomes, and the use of angiotensin-converting enzyme inhibitors. Am J Med 2000;109:605–13.

[34] Pernenkil R, Vinson JM, Shah AS, et al. Course and prognosis in patients > or = 70 years of age with congestive heart failure and normal versus abnormal left ventricular ejection fraction. Am J Cardiol 1997;79:216–9.

[35] McDermott MM, Feinglass J, Lee PI, et al. Systolic function, readmission rates, and survival among consecutively hospitalized patients with congestive heart failure. Am Heart J 1997;134:728–36.

[36] Vasan RS, Larson MG, Benjamin EJ, et al. Congestive heart failure in subjects with normal versus reduced left ventricular ejection fraction: prevalence and mortality in a population-based cohort. J Am Coll Cardiol 1999;33:1948–55.

[37] McAlister FA, Teo KK, Taher M, et al. Insights into the contemporary epidemiology and outpatient management of congestive heart failure. Am Heart J 1999;138:87–94.

[38] Senni M, Tribouilloy CM, Rodeheffer RJ, et al. Congestive heart failure in the community: a study of all incident cases in Olmsted County, Minnesota, in 1991. Circulation 1998;98:2282–9.

[39] Rich MW, McSherry F, Williford WO, et al. Effect of age on mortality, hospitalizations and response to digoxin in patients with heart failure: the DIG Study. J Am Coll Cardiol 2001;38:806–13.

[40] Tarantini L, Faggiano P, Senni M, et al. Clinical features and prognosis associated with a preserved left ventricular systolic function in a large cohort of congestive heart failure outpatients managed by cardiologists: data from the Italian Network on Congestive Heart Failure. Ital Heart J 2002;3: 656–64.

[41] The Digitalis Investigation Group. The effect of digoxin on mortality and morbidity in patients with heart failure. N Engl J Med 1997;336:525–33.

[42] Judge KW, Pawitan Y, Caldwell J, et al. Congestive heart failure symptoms in patients with preserved left ventricular systolic function: analysis of the CASS registry. J Am Coll Cardiol 1991; 18:377–82.

[43] Bonow RO, Udelson JE. Left ventricular diastolic dysfunction as a cause of congestive heart failure: mechanisms and management. Ann Intern Med 1992;117:502–10.

[44] McDonald IG. The shape and movements of the human left ventricle during systole: a study by cineangiography and by cineradiography of epicardial markers. Am J Cardiol 1970;26:221–30.

[45] Ingels NB, Daughters GT, Stinson EB, et al. Measurement of midwall myocardial dynamics in intact man by radiography of surgically implanted markers. Circulation 1975;52:859–67.

[46] Rothfeld JM, LeWinter MM, Tischler MD. Left ventricular systolic torsion and early diastolic filling by echocardiography in normal humans. Am J Cardiol 1998;81:1465–9.

[47] Michelfelder EC, Khoury P, Witt SA, et al. Noncircumferential myofiber function: impact on early diastolic filling in children. J Am Soc Echocardiogr 2001;14:1065–9.

[48] Rademakers FE, Buchalter MB, Rogers WJ, et al. Dissociation between left ventricular untwisting and filling: accentuation by catecholamines. Circulation 1992;85:1572–81.

[49] Udelson JE, Bacharach SL, Cannon RO III, et al. Minimum left ventricular pressure during beta-adrenergic stimulation in human subjects: evidence for elastic recoil and diastolic "suction" in the normal heart. Circulation 1990;82:1174–82.

[50] Zile MR, Brutsaert DL. New concepts in diastolic dysfunction and diastolic heart failure II. Causal mechanisms and treatment. Circulation 2002;105: 1503–8.

[51] Nayler WG, Poole-Wilson PA, Williams A. Hypoxia and calcium. J Mol Cell Cardiol 1979;11: 683–706.

[52] Henry PD, Schuchleib R, Davis J, et al. Myocardial contracture and accumulation of mitochondrial calcium in ischemic rabbit heart. Am J Physiol 1977;233:H677–84.

[53] Weisfeldt ML, Armstrong P, Scully HE, et al. Incomplete relaxation between beats after myocardial hypoxia and ischemia. J Clin Invest 1974;53: 1626–36.

[54] Sordahl LA, McCollum WB, Wood WG, et al. Mitochondria and sarcoplasmic reticulum function in cardiac hypertrophy and failure. Am J Physiol 1973;224:497–502.

[55] Ito Y, Suko J, Chidsey CA. Intracellular calcium and myocardial contractility. V. Calcium uptake of sarcoplasmic reticulum fractions in hypertrophied and failing rabbit hearts. J Mol Cell Cardiol 1974;6:237–47.

[56] Gwathmey JK, Copelas L, MacKinnon R, et al. Abnormal intracellular calcium handling in myocardium from patients with end-stage heart failure. Circ Res 1987;61:70–6.

[57] Bell SP, Nyland L, Tischler MD, et al. Alterations in the determinants of diastolic suction during pacing tachycardia. Circ Res 2000;87:235–40.

[58] Cazorla O, Freiburg A, Helmes M, et al. Differential expression of cardiac titin isoforms and modulation of cellular stiffness. Circ Res 2000;86:59–67.

[59] Jalil JE, Doering CW, Janicki JS, et al. Fibrillar collagen and myocardial stiffness in the intact hypertrophied rat left ventricle. Circ Res 1989;64: 1041–50.

[60] Weber KT, Janicki JS, Pick R, et al. Myocardial fibrosis and pathologic hypertrophy in the rat with renovascular hypertension. Am J Cardiol 1990;65: G1–7.

[61] Kato S, Spinale FG, Tanaka R, et al. Inhibition of collagen cross-linking: effects on fibrillar collagen and ventricular diastolic function. Am J Physiol 1995;269:H863–8.

[62] Raman VK, Lee YA, Lindpaintner K. The cardiac renin-angiotensin-aldosterone system and hypertensive cardiac hypertrophy. Am J Cardiol 1995; 76:18D–23D.

[63] Dzau VJ. Tissue renin-angiotensin system in myocardial hypertrophy and failure. Arch Intern Med 1993;153:937–42.

[64] Schunkert H, Dzau VJ, Tang SS, et al. Increased rat cardiac angiotensin converting enzyme activity and mRNA expression in pressure overload left ventricular hypertrophy: effects on coronary resistance, contractility and relaxation. J Clin Invest 1990;86: 1913–20.

[65] Eberli FR, Apstein CS, Ngoy S, et al. Exacerbation of left ventricular ischemic diastolic dysfunction by pressure-overload hypertrophy: modification by specific inhibition of cardiac angiotensin converting enzyme. Circ Res 1992;70:931 43.

[66] Mochizuki T, Eberli FR, Apstein CS, et al. Exacerbation of ischemic dysfunction by angiotensin II in red cell-perfused rabbit hearts: Effects of coronary flow, contractility, and high-energy phosphate metabolism. J Clin Invest 1992;89:490–8.

[67] Zennaro MC, Farman N, Bonbalet JP, et al. Tissue-specific expression of alpha and beta messenger ribonucleic acid isoforms of the human mineralocorticoid receptor in normal and pathological states. J Clin Endocrinol Metab 1997;82: 1345–52.

[68] Weber KT. Aldosterone in congestive heart failure. N Engl J Med 2001;345:1689–97.

[69] Horisberger JD, Rossier BC. Aldosterone regulation of gene transcription leading to control of ion transport. Hypertension 1992;19:221 7.

[70] Robert V, Van Thiem N, Cheav SL, et al. Increased cardiac types I and III collagen mRNAs in aldosterone-salt hypertension. Hypertension 1994;24: 30–6.

[71] Khan NU, Movahed A. The role of aldosterone and aldosterone-receptor antagonists in heart failure. Rev Cardiovasc Med 2004;5:71–81.

[72] Laine GA. Microvascular changes in the heart during chronic arterial hypertension. Circ Res 1988;62: 953–60.

[73] White M, Leenen FH. Aging and cardiovascular responsiveness to beta-agonist in humans: role of changes in beta-receptor responses versus baroreflex activity. Clin Pharmacol Ther 1994;56:543–53.

[74] Lakatta EG, Yin FC. Myocardial aging: functional alterations and related cellular mechanisms. Am J Physiol 1982;242:H927–41.

[75] O'Rourke MF. Diastolic heart failure, diastolic left ventricular dysfunction and exercise intolerance. J Am Coll Cardiol 2001;38:803–5.

[76] Lamb HJ, Beyerbacht HP, van der Laarse A, et al. Diastolic dysfunction in hypertensive heart disease is associated with altered myocardial metabolism. Circulation 1999;99:2261–7.

[77] Zhang J, McDonald KM. Bioenergetic consequences of left ventricular remodeling. Circulation 1995;92:1011–9.

[78] Yelamarty RV, Moore RL, Yu FT, et al. Relaxation abnormalities in single cardiac myocytes from renovascular hypertensive rats. Am J Physiol 1992;262:C980–90.

[79] Leite-Moreira AF, Correia-Pinto J, Gillebert TC. Afterload induced changes in myocardial relaxation: a mechanism for diastolic dysfunction. Cardiovasc Res 1999;43:344–53.

[80] Sadoshima J, Xu Y, Slayter HS, et al. Autocrine release of angiotensin II mediates stretch-induced hypertrophy of cardiac myocytes in vitro. Cell 1993; 75:977–84.

[81] Van Heugten HA, De Jonge HW, Bezstarosti K, et al. Intracellular signaling and genetic reprogramming during agonist-induced hypertrophy of cardiomyocytes. Ann N Y Acad Sci 1995;752:343–52.

[82] Poulsen SH, Jensen SE, Egstrup K. Longitudinal changes and prognostic implications of left ventricular diastolic function in first acute myocardial infarction. Am Heart J 1999;137.910–8.

[83] Pardaens K, Van Cleemput J, Vanhaecke J, et al. Atrial fibrillation is associated with a lower exercise capacity in male chronic heart failure patients. Heart 1997;78:564–8.

[84] Gottdiener JS, Arnold AM, Aurigemma GP, et al. Predictors of congestive heart failure in the elderly: the Cardiovascular Health Study. J Am Coll Cardiol 2000;35:1628–37.

[85] Parker AB, Yusuf S, Naylor CD. The relevance of subgroup-specific treatment effects: the Studies of Left Ventricular Dysfunction (SOLVD) revisited. Am Heart J 2002;144:941–7.

[86] Arnold JM, Yusuf S, Young J, et al. Prevention of heart failure in patients in the Heart Outcomes Prevention Evaluation (HOPE) study. Circulation 2003;107:1284–90.

[87] Seneviratne BI. Diabetic cardiomyopathy: the preclinical phase. BMJ 1977;1:1444 6.

[88] Raev DC. Which left ventricular function is impaired earlier in the evolution of diabetic cardiomyopathy?: an echocardiographic study of young type I diabetic patients. Diabetes Care 1994;17:633–9.

[89] Zabalgoitia M, Ismaeil MF, Anderson L, et al. Prevalence of diastolic dysfunction in normotensive, asymptomatic patients with well-controlled type 2 diabetes mellitus. Am J Cardiol 2001;87: 320–3.

[90] Liu JE, Palmieri V, Roman MJ, et al. The impact of diabetes on left ventricular filling pattern in

normotensive and hypertensive adults: the Strong Heart Study. J Am Coll Cardiol 2001;37:1943–9.

[91] Uusitupa M, Siitonen O, Aro A, et al. Effect of correction of hyperglycemia on left ventricular function in non-insulin-dependent (type 2) diabetics. Acta Med Scand 1983;213:363–8.

[92] Hardin N. The myocardial and vascular pathology of diabetic cardiomyopathy. Coron Artery Dis 1996;7:99–108.

[93] Young ME, McNulty P, Taegtmeyer H. Adaptation and maladaptation of the heart in diabetes. II. Potential mechanisms. Circulation 2002;105:1861–70.

[94] Rupp H, Elimban V, Dhalla NS. Modification of myosin isozymes and SR Ca(2 +)-pump ATPase of the diabetic rat heart by lipid-lowering interventions. Mol Cell Biochem 1994;132:69–80.

[95] Bristow MR. Why does the myocardium fail?: insights from basic science. Lancet 1998;352:S8–14.

[96] Depre C, Young ME, Ying J, et al. Streptozotocin-induced changes in cardiac gene expression in the absence of severe contractile dysfunction. J Mol Cell Cardiol 2000;32:985–96.

[97] Golfman L, Dixon IM, Takeda N, et al. Differential changes in cardiac myofibrillar and sarcoplasmic reticular gene expression in alloxan-induced diabetes. Mol Cell Biochem 1999;200:15–25.

[98] Flarsheim CE, Grupp IL, Matlib MA. Mitochondrial dysfunction accompanies diastolic dysfunction in diabetic rat heart. Am J Physiol 1996;271: H192–202.

[99] Bristow M. Etomoxir: a new approach to treatment of chronic heart failure. Lancet 2000;356:1621–2.

[100] Yusuf S, Pfeffer MA, Swedberg K, et al. Effects of candesartan in patients with chronic HF and preserved left-ventricular ejection fraction: the CHARM-Preserved Trial. Lancet 2003;362: 777–81.

[101] Officers ALLHAT and Coordinators for the ALLHAT Collaborative Research Group. Major outcomes in high-risk hypertensive patients randomized to angiotensin-converting enzyme inhibitor or calcium channel blocker vs diuretic: the Antihypertensive and Lipid-Lowering Treatment to Prevent Heart Attack Trial (ALLHAT). JAMA 2002;288:2981–97.

[102] The Heart Outcomes Prevention Evaluation Investigators. Effects of an angiotensin-converting-enzyme inhibitor, ramipril, on cardiovascular events in high-risk patients. N Engl J Med 2000; 342:145–53.

[103] Lonn EM, Yusuf S, Jha P, et al. Emerging role of angiotensin-converting enzyme inhibitors in cardiac and vascular protection. Circulation 1994;90: 2056–69.

[104] Schieffer B, Schieffer E, Hilfiker-Kleiner D, et al. Expression of angiotensin II and interleukin 6 in human coronary atherosclerotic plaques: potential implications for inflammation and plaque instability. Circulation 2000;101:1372–8.

[105] The European trial on reduction of cardiac events with perindopril in stable coronary artery disease Investigators. Efficacy of perindopril in reduction of cardiovascular events among patients with stable coronary artery disease: randomised, double-blind, placebo-controlled, multicentre trial (the EUROPA study). Lancet 2003;362:782–8.

[106] Pedersen OD, Bagger H, Kober L, et al. Trandolapril reduces the incidence of atrial fibrillation after acute myocardial infarction in patients with left ventricular dysfunction. Circulation 1999;100: 376–80.

[107] Vermes E, Tardif JC, Bourassa MG, et al. Enalapril decreases the incidence of atrial fibrillation in patients with left ventricular dysfunction: insight from the Studies Of Left Ventricular Dysfunction (SOLVD) trials. Circulation 2003;10:2926–31.

[108] Hansson L, Lindholm LH, Niskanen L, et al. Effect of angiotensin-converting- enzyme inhibition compared with conventional therapy on cardiovascular morbidity and mortality in hypertension: the Captopril Prevention Project (CAPPP) randomised trial. Lancet 1999;353:611–6.

[109] Pitt B, Reichek N, Willenbrock R, et al. Effects of eplerenone, enalapril, and eplerenone/enalapril in patients with essential hypertension and left ventricular hypertrophy. The 4E-left ventricular hypertrophy study. Circulation 2003;108: 1831–8.

[110] Brilla CG, Funck RC, Rupp H. Lisionpril-mediated regression of myocardial fibrosis in patients with hypertensive heart disease. Circulation 2000; 102:1388–93.

[111] Julius S, Kjeldsen SE, Weber M, et al, for the VALUE trial group. Outcomes in hypertensive patients at high cardiovascular risk treated with regimens based on valsartan or amlodipine: the VALUE randomised trial. Lancet 2004;363: 2022–31.

[112] Dahlof B, Devereux RB, Kjeldsen SE, et al, for the LIFE Study Group. Cardiovascular morbidity and mortality in the Losartan Intervention For Endpoint reduction in hypertension study (LIFE): a randomised trial against atenolol. Lancet 2002; 359:995–1003.

[113] Lithell H, Hansson L, Skoog I, et al. The Study on Cognition and Prognosis in the Elderly (SCOPE): principal results of a randomized double-blind intervention trial. J Hypertens 2003;21:875–86.

[114] Madrid AH, Bueno MG, Rebollo JM, et al. Use of irbesartan to maintain sinus rhythm in patients with long-lasting persistent atrial fibrillation: a prospective and randomized study. Circulation 2002; 106:331–6.

[115] Devereux RB, Gerdts E, Wachtell K, et al. Regression of hypertensive left ventricular hypertrophy by angiotensin receptor blockade versus beta-blockade: the LIFE trial (abstract). Am J Hypertens 2002;15:15A.

[116] Coope J, Warrender TS. Randomised trial of treatment of hypertension in elderly patients in primary care. BMJ 1986;293:1145–51.

[117] Ekbom T, Dahlof B, Hansson L, et al. Antihypertensive efficacy and side effects of three beta-blockers and a diuretic in elderly hypertensives: a report from the STOP-Hypertension study. J Hypertens 1992;10:1525–30.

[118] MRC Working Party. Medical Research Council trial of treatment of hypertension in older adults: principal results. BMJ 1992;304:405–12.

[119] Messerli F, Grossman E. Beta-blockers in hypertension: is carvedilol different? Am J Cardiol 2004;93(Suppl):7B–12B.

[120] Norwegian Multicenter Study Group. Timolol-induced reduction in mortality and reinfarction in patients surviving acute myocardial infarction. N Engl J Med 1981;304:801–7.

[121] Beta-Blocker Heart Attack Trial Research Group. A randomized trial of propranolol in patients with acute myocardial infarction: I. Mortality results. JAMA 1982;247:1707–14.

[122] Beta-Blocker Heart Attack Trial Research Group. A randomized trial of propranolol in patients with acute myocardial infarction: II. Morbidity results. JAMA 1983;250:2814–9.

[123] Vantrimpont P, Rouleau JL, Wun CC, et al. Additive beneficial effects of beta-blockers to angiotensin-converting enzyme inhibitors in the Survival and Ventricular Enlargement (SAVE) Study. SAVE Investigators. J Am Coll Cardiol 1997;29:229–36.

[124] Spargias KS, Hall AS, Greenwood DC, et al. Beta-blocker treatment and other prognostic variables in patients with clinical evidence of heart failure after acute myocardial infarction: evidence from the AIRE study. Heart 1999;81:25–32.

[125] Wyse DG, Waldo AL, DiMarco JP, et al. A comparison of rate control and rhythm control in patients with atrial fibrillation. N Engl J Med 2002;347:1825–33.

[126] Olshansky B, Rosenfeld LE, Warner AL, et al. The Atrial Fibrillation Follow-Up Investigation of Rhythm Management (AFFIRM) study approaches to control rate in atrial fibrillation. J Am Coll Cardiol 2004;43:1201–8.

[127] Kuhlkamp V, Schirdewan A, Stangl K, et al. Use of metoprolol CR/XL to maintain sinus rhythm after conversion from persistent atrial fibrillation: a randomized, double-blind, placebo-controlled study. J Am Coll Cardiol 2000;36:139–46.

[128] Schmieder RE, Schlaich MP, Klingbeil AU, et al. Update on reversal of left ventricular hypertrophy in essential hypertension (a meta-analysis of all randomized double-blind studies until December 1996). Nephrol Dial Transplant 1998;13:564–9.

[129] Palazzuoli A, Carrera A, Calabria P, et al. Effects of carvedilol therapy on restrictive diastolic filling pattern in chronic heart failure. Am Heart J 2004;147:1–7.

[130] Capomolla S, Febo O, Gnemmi M, et al. Beta-blockade therapy in chronic heart failure: diastolic function and mitral regurgitation improvement by carvedilol. Am Heart J 2000;139:596–608.

[131] Bergstrom A, Andersson B, Edner M, et al. Effect of carvedilol on diastolic function in patients with diastolic heart failure and preserved systolic function. Results of the Swedish Doppler-echocardiographic study (SWEDIC). Eur J Heart Fail 2004;6:453–61.

[132] Taylor CT. Eplerenone (Inspra) for hypertension. Am Fam Physician 2004;69:915–6.

[133] Williams GH, Burgess E, Kolloch RE, et al. Efficacy of eplerenone versus enalapril as monotherapy in systemic hypertension. Am J Cardiol 2004;93:990–6.

[134] White WB, Duprez D, St. Hillaire R, et al. Effects of the selective aldosterone blocker eplerenone versus the calcium antagonist amlodipine in systolic hypertension. Hypertension 2003;41:1021–6.

[135] Flack JM, Oparil S, Pratt JH, et al. Efficacy and tolerability of eplerenone and losartan in hypertensive black and white patients. J Am Coll Cardiol 2003;41:1148–55.

[136] Robert V, Heymes C, Silvestre JS, et al. Angiotensin AT1 receptor subtype as a cardiac target of aldosterone: role in aldosterone-salt induced fibrosis. Hypertension 1999;33:981–6.

[137] Duprez DA, DeBuyzere ML, Rietzschel ER, et al. Inverse relationship between aldosterone and large artery compliance in chronically treated heart failure patients. Eur Heart J 1998;19:1371–6.

[138] Bauersachs J, Heck M, Fraccarollo D, et al. Addition of spironolactone to angiotensin-converting enzyme inhibition in heart failure improves endothelial vasomotor dysfunction: role of vascular superoxide anion formation and endothelial nitric oxide synthase expression. J Am Coll Cardiol 2002;39:351–8.

[139] Brilla CG, Matsubara LS, Weber KT. Antifibrotic effects of spironolactone in preventing myocardial fibrosis in systemic arterial hypertension. Am J Cardiol 1993;71:12A–6A.

[140] Brilla CG, Matsubara LS, Weber KT. Anti-aldosterone treatment and prevention of myocardial fibrosis in primary and secondary hyperaldosteronism. J Mol Cell Cardiol 1993;25:563–75.

[141] Lacolley P, Safar ME, Lucet B, et al. Prevention of aortic and cardiac fibrosis by spironolactone in old normotensive rats. J Am Coll Cardiol 2001;37:662–7.

[142] Zannad F, Alla F, Dousset B, et al. Limitation of excessive extracellular matrix turnover may contribute to survival benefit of spironolactone therapy in patients with congestive heart failure. Circulation 2000;102:2700–6.

[143] Querejeta R, Varo N, Lopez B, et al. Serum car-
boxy-terminal propeptide of procollagen type I is
a marker of myocardial fibrosis in hypertensive
heart disease. Circulation 2000;101:1729–35.

[144] Frierdich G, Schuh J, Brown M, et al. Effects of the
selective mineralocorticoid receptor antagonist,
eplerenone, in a model of aldosterone-induced hypertension and cardiac fibrosis [abstract]. Am
J Hypertens 1998;11:94.

[145] Suzuki G, Morita H, Mishima T, et al. Effects of
long-term monotherapy with eplerenone, a novel
aldosterone blocker, on progression of left ventricular dysfunction and remodeling in dogs with heart
failure. Circulation 2002;106:2967–72.

[146] Struthers AD, MacDonald TM. Review of aldoste-
rone- and angiotensin II-induced target organ damage and prevention. Cardiovasc Res 2004;61:
663–70.

[147] Shepherd J, Cobbe SM, Ford I, et al. Prevention of
coronary heart disease with pravastatin in men with
hypercholesterolemia. West of Scotland Coronary
Prevention Study Group. N Engl J Med 1995;333:
1301–7.

[148] Heart Protection Study Collaborative Group.
MRC/BHF Heart Protection Study of cholesterol
lowering with simvastatin in 20,536 high-risk individuals: a randomised placebo-controlled trial.
Lancet 2002;360:7–22.

[149] Randomised trial of cholesterol lowering in 4444
patients with coronary heart disease: the Scandinavian Simvastatin Survival Study (4S). Lancet 1994;
344:1383–9.

[150] Sacks FM, Pfeffer MA, Moye LA, et al. The effect
of pravastatin on coronary events after myocardial
infarction in patients with average cholesterol
levels. Cholesterol and Recurrent Events Trial investigators. N Engl J Med 1996;335:1001–9.

[151] Prevention of cardiovascular events and death with
pravastatin in patients with coronary heart disease
and a broad range of initial cholesterol levels. The
Long-Term Intervention with Pravastatin in
Ischaemic Disease (LIPID) Study Group. N Engl
J Med 1998;339:1349–57.

[152] Iribarren C, Karter AJ, Go AS, et al. Glycemic control and heart failure among adult patients with
diabetes. Circulation 2001;103:2668–73.

Neutral Endopeptidase Inhibitors and Endothelin Antagonists

Srinivas Iyengar, MD[a],*, William T. Abraham, MD, FACP, FACC[b]

[a]Columbia University Medical Center, New York, NY, USA
[b]Ohio State University, Columbus, OH, USA

Over the last 15 years, the deleterious effects of the neurohormonal cascade on the failing heart have been documented increasingly. Treatment algorithms for patients who have systolic heart failure revolve around offsetting the effects of this hormonal barrage. The use of angiotensin-converting enzyme (ACE) inhibitors [1], beta-blockers [2], aldosterone antagonists [3], and angiotensin II–receptor blockers [4] have formed the cornerstone of heart failure therapy. Using this theory of hormonal antagonism, additional therapeutic agents have been developed. Two newer classes, neutral endopeptidase (NEP) inhibitors and endothelin (ET) antagonists, are medications that showed promise in initial studies, but, as a possible indication that the pathoetiology of heart failure is more complex than is understood, larger clinical trials with these agents fell short of expected results.

Neutral endopeptidase inhibitors

Background

NEP is a membrane-bound metallopeptidase that functions to cleave endogenous peptides at the amino side of hydrophilic residues [5]. NEP is found in various cell lines, including endothelial cells and vascular smooth muscle cells [6,7], as well as in various organs. Natriuretic hormones, such as atrial natriuretic peptide, brain natriuretic peptide, and C-type natriuretic peptide, are peptides whose degradation is facilitated by the actions of NEP [8,9]. In addition, NEP catalyzes the degradation of endothelin-1 (ET-1) and angiotensin II [10]. NEP inhibitors, as their name suggests, counteract the functions of NEP. This dual antagonism of the degradation process for vasoconstrictive and vasodilatory peptides has led to questions about how NEP inhibition affects the vascular system given its effects on these two seemingly opposite entities.

Experimental data

This idea of nonselective (between constrictive versus dilatory peptides) degradation inhibition has resulted in studies with mixed conclusions about which action is predominant in NEP inhibition. Studies examining patients who have essential hypertension have shown improvement and worsening during treatment with NEP inhibitors [11,12]; it is theorized that the response to NEP inhibition is linked to the amounts of predominant substrate present, whether vasoconstrictive or vasodilatory. This could explain why NEP inhibitors have shown beneficial hemodynamic effects in hypertensive patients but not in normotensive patients [13].

In the area of heart failure, NEP inhibitors have had varying results. Although Kahn and colleagues [14] demonstrated the natriuretic effects of NEP inhibition with the lowering of pulmonary capillary wedge pressure (PCWP) and Good and colleagues [15] showed a dose-dependent diuresis with candoxatrilat in moderate to severe heart

A version of this article originally appeared in *Heart Failure Clinics*, volume 1, issue 1.

* Corresponding author. Division of Cardiology, Columbia University Medical Center, 630 West 168th Street, New York, NY 10032.

E-mail address: sri9002@nyp.org (S. Iyengar).

failure patients, chronic treatment with these medications has not produced similar results.

Recently, several trials have investigated a modified form of NEP inhibitor: the vasopeptidase inhibitors. These compounds are composed of dual metalloprotease inhibitors that simultaneously block ACE and NEP. The drive for this new therapeutic agent stemmed from the idea that these agents together could have a beneficial synergistic effect on vascular hemodynamics and renal function not seen with individual use [16,17].

Several vasopeptide inhibitors have been studied, in small animal and human models, and the initial results were particularly favorable regarding the treatment of hypertension [18,19]. The most thoroughly studied vasopeptide inhibitor, omapatrilat, had a beneficial effect on blood pressure in hypertensive rats [20] as well as in heart-failure hamster models, even compared with an ACE inhibitor [21]. Although many of the clinical trials in which omapatrilat was used were in the antihypertensive arena, it also was examined for potential use in heart failure.

McClean and colleagues [22] published data on a study of 48 patients who had New York Heart Association (NYHA) class-II to -III heart failure treated with omapatrilat who reported improvement in functional class, as well as increases in left ventricular function. These data were bolstered by the IMPRESS trial [23], which sought to determine the long-term effects of omapatrilat on exercise tolerance and morbidity compared with lisinopril. Five hundred seventy-three patients who had NYHA class-II to -IV chronic heart failure were assigned randomly to receive either omapatrilat at a target dose of 40 mg/d or lisinopril at a target dose of 20 mg/d for 24 weeks, with the primary endpoints focusing on improvement in exercise tolerance at week 12. Secondary endpoints such as death and comorbid events indicative of worsening heart failure also were examined. At week 12, no significant difference in exercise tolerance was seen between the two groups. At the end of the study, there were no statistical differences between omapatrilat and lisinopril in the frequencies of death or hospitalization, but omapatrilat significantly decreased the composite endpoint of death, hospitalization, or discontinuation of study treatment for worsening heart failure compared with lisinopril (6% versus 10%, $P = .035$). Improvement in NYHA functional class also was related more closely to omapatrilat than to lisinopril therapy.

The largest trial investigating omapatrilat's role in heart failure was the Omapatrilat Versus Enalapril Randomized Trial of Utility in Reducing Events (OVERTURE) trial, which randomized 5770 patients who had NYHA class-II to -IV heart failure to either omapatrilat, 40 mg, or an uptitrated dose of enalapril, 10 mg twice daily [24]. Primary endpoints (death or hospitalization for chronic heart failure requiring intravenous medication) were not significantly different between the drugs (Table 1). In addition, there was an increased incidence of hypotension, dizziness, cough, and angioedema with omapatrilat therapy compared with patients treated with enalapril, although impaired renal function and fatigue were seen more frequently in the enalapril arm (Table 2). A post hoc analysis, however, which defined hospitalization for heart failure as any hospitalization for heart failure requiring a change in regimen, whether oral or intravenous, showed omapatrilat to be superior to enalapril. In subgroup analyses, an advantage of omapatrilat over enalapril was found among women, those who had hypertension (systolic pressure > 140 mm Hg) at the start of the study, and those without diabetes mellitus. Among patients who had pre-existing hypertension, the incidence of renal impairment was lower for the omapatrilat group (3.9% versus 7.1%).

McClean and colleagues [25] followed up their initial work with a study investigating different dosing regimens of omapatrilat. In a randomized, double-blind, multicenter trial, 369 patients who had NYHA class II- to IV heart failure and ejection fractions of less than 40% were assigned randomly to receive 12 weeks of omapatrilat, 2.5 to 40 mg/d, as a replacement to ACE inhibitor therapy. ACE inhibitors were discontinued at least 4 days before randomization. Hemodynamic and neurohormonal parameters were evaluated at

Table 1
Overture trial results

Endpoint	Enalapril n = 2884	Omapatrilat n = 2886	P value
Primary			
Death and/or HF hospitalization	973	914	.187
Secondary			
All-cause mortality	509	477	.339
CV death and/or CV hospitalization	1275	1178	.024

Abbreviations: CV, cardiovascular; HF, heart failure.

Table 2
Overture trial adverse events

Event	Enalapril n = 2884 (%)	Omapatrilat n = 2886 (%)
Dizziness	401 (13.9)	561 (19.4)
Hyportension	332 (11.5)	564 (19.5)
Renal impairment	291 (10.1)	196 (6.8)
Fatigue	276 (9.6)	233 (8.1)
Cough	259 (9.0)	279 (9.7)
Angioedema	14 (0.5)	24 (0.8)

baseline and at the end of the study. Treatment with omapatrilat resulted in a dose-related reduction of PCWP, systolic and diastolic blood pressure, and systemic vascular resistance. In addition, a dose-dependent increase in left ventricular ejection fraction was reported, but no significant changes in cardiac index were noted. On a neurohormonal level, treatment with omapatrilat resulted in decreased NEP activity, whereas no significant changes in trough plasma epinephrine, norepinephrine, or ET-1 levels were seen during treatment. In addition, improvement in NYHA functional class correlated more strongly with patients being treated with higher dosages of omapatrilat. Despite the encouraging data, the initial results of the OVERTURE trial loom large, and the debate over the applicability of using vasopeptide inhibitors to treat heart failure continues.

Discussion

There are three main theories for NEP inhibition alone and its lack of clinical efficacy for heart failure: (1) the dual inhibition of peptide degradation by NEP inhibitors can increase disproportionately the activity of the renin-angiotensin-aldosterone system (RAAS) and ET over time, (2) tolerance to natriuretic peptides might develop with chronic treatment, and (3) down-regulation of natriuretic peptide receptors in response to the decreased degradation of natriuretic peptides may be a factor. Alone or in combination, these theories could explain the lack of clinical benefit seen with these agents.

NEP and ACE-inhibition combinations have not been demonstrated more effective than other standard agents for treating heart failure. Omapatrilat, the vasopeptidase inhibitor most extensively studied, did not demonstrate any incremental benefit over ACE inhibition alone, and had more side effects in relation to

angioedema [24]. There are two possible explanations: (1) these results could be limited to the actions of omapatrilat, not all vasopeptidase inhibitors and (2) the effects of bradykinin. Although bradykinin can be related to the positive effects of ACE inhibitors by accentuating some of their blood pressure–reducing actions, too much bradykinin (through NEP and ACE inhibition) may tip the scales in the opposite direction. The end result might be the best explanation for the increase in angioedema seen with vasopeptide inhibitor use [26].

Although there may be several factors responsible for omapatrilat's failure to distinguish itself as a superior or equal therapy to ACE inhibitors, it has widened the knowledge base of researchers focused on the development of hormone-specific therapies for heart failure.

Endothelin antagonists

Background

ET is a 21–amino acid peptide that is produced by endopeptidase cleavage of preproendothelin [27]. Yanagisawa [28] first described it in 1988 as an exceptionally potent vasoconstrictor. Various types of cells in the heart, lung, and other organs produce ET [29]. ET-1 to -4 are produced from big ET by an ET-converting enzyme. The formation of ET is stimulated by cytokines, catecholamines, and hormones, as well as by vasoactive agents [30,31]. The effects of ET include vasoconstriction of vascular smooth muscle, increased production of cardiac fibroblasts, and hypertrophy of cardiac myocytes [32]. Furthermore, in patients with intact cardiac function, ET seems to have a positive inotropic effect, although its inotropic effect in heart failure is questionable [33]. ET has been associated with two main receptor types: type A (ET-A) and type B (ET-B) [34]. ET-A receptor has been associated with potent vasoconstriction and cell hypertrophy, whereas ET-B receptor has been associated with more vasodilatory effects, although its exact role is not known. Elevated serum levels of ET have been found in patients who have decompensated heart failure, and these levels have been associated with negative clinical parameters and poorer overall prognosis [35–37]. With the consequences of the pathologic effects of ET increasingly being realized, creating agents that could inhibit the production of ET or antagonize its ability to interact with its receptors was appealing. After the introduction of ET-receptor antagonists for the treatment of pulmonary hypertension [38], it was believed to be only a matter of time before the indications of these agents would be extended to heart failure.

Experimental data

ET-receptor antagonists first were investigated in various animal models of heart failure. Sakai and colleagues [39] demonstrated that long-term treatment with a selective ET-A receptor antagonist in the treatment of post–myocardial infarction heart failure rat models could decrease mortality and increase ventricular function. Studies using nonselective ET-receptor antagonists with the same type of rat model have demonstrated similar results [40]. Although early administration (within 3–6 hours) of an ET-receptor antagonist, selective or nonselective, post–myocardial infarction has been associated with increased left ventricular dysfunction and mortality in animal models [41,42], the weight of positive evidence from additional animal studies pointed to an overall favorable effect of these agents for the treatment of heart failure [43–45]. The beneficial effects of ET-receptor antagonists in animal models initially were demonstrated using intravenous formulations, but these effects also were seen with oral preparations [46].

Although bolstered by the strength of several experimental animal trials, researchers still questioned: how would ET antagonists fare in the human heart failure population? Small, short-term trials examining the use of ET antagonists in patients who had heart failure were initially promising [47,48]. These first results encouraged larger studies. The effect of long-term bosentan use on the primary endpoint of all-cause mortality or hospitalization for heart failure was examined in the Research on Endothelin Antagonist in Chronic Heart Failure (REACH-1) study, which revealed improvements in reducing the combined endpoints of death and worsening heart failure after 6 months, but was associated with an increase in liver enzymes [49]. In addition, bosentan was associated with more heart failure events during the first 6 months. This study was conducted with a bosentan dose of 500 mg twice daily, and it was believed that the elevated enzymes were a dose-dependent phenomenon.

This trial was followed by the Endothelin Antagonist Bosentan for Lowering Cardiac Events in Heart Failure (ENABLE) study, which used a lower dose of bosentan, 125 mg twice daily, in patients who had NYHA class-IIIB to -IV heart failure [50]. Despite fewer adverse enzyme interactions than in the REACH-1 study, no overall mortality benefit was revealed with this therapy. The Heart Failure ET-A Receptor Blockade Trial examined the effects of darusentan, a selective ET-A receptor antagonist, in 157 NYHA class-II heart failure patients. Patients were treated for 3 weeks, and certain hemodynamic parameters (cardiac output, systemic vascular resistance) improved, but others (PCWP) did not change significantly [51].

The Randomized Intravenous Tezosentan (RITZ) study groups examined the hemodynamic and clinical effects of tezosentan, a nonselective ET-receptor antagonist, for the treatment of heart failure. Although RITZ-2 demonstrated an improvement in cardiac index and lowering of PCWP compared with placebo [52], RITZ-1 failed to demonstrate any difference in the primary endpoint of change in dyspnea compared with placebo [53]. In addition, RITZ-4 revealed that treatment with tezosentan did not improve significantly any of the major clinical endpoints, including death or worsening heart failure [54]. RITZ-5 evaluated oxygen saturations in patients who had heart failure and pulmonary edema and found no significant difference between the placebo and medication arms [55].

The Enrasentan Clinical Outcomes Randomized (ENCORE) study compared the nonselective ET-receptor antagonist enrasentan (at varying doses) with placebo or high-dose ACE inhibition for 9 months in 419 patients who had NYHA class-II or -III heart failure [52]. Negative trends seen with the enrasentan arm included worsening heart failure and excess mortality (Fig. 1).

The Endothelin-A Receptor Antagonist Trial in Heart Failure (EARTH) trial examined the effects of darusentan (at varying doses) compared with placebo in NYHA class-II to -IV heart failure patients who also had depressed ejection fractions and were on stable oral heart failure therapy [56]. The primary endpoint of the study was the effect these therapies had on left ventricular remodeling, as determined by cardiac MRI; in addition, 6-minute walk tests and quality-of-life assessments were performed. Although there was a weak positive trend for darusentan at higher doses for reduction of left ventricular end-systolic volumes, it was not statistically significant. It also was reported that darusentan did not reduce the incidence of death, all-cause hospitalizations, or

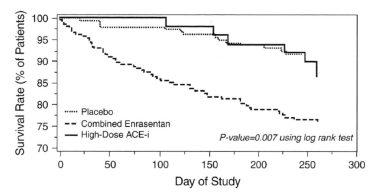

Fig. 1. Results of the ENCORE Trial showing time to death, heart failure hospitalization, or withdrawal caused by worsening heart failure. ACE-I, ACE inhibitor. (*Data from* Abraham WT. Results of the ENCORE Trial. Presented at: Scientific Sessions of the American College of Cardiology, 2001.)

hospitalizations caused by heart failure. No significant differences between placebo and darusentan in relation to the 6-minute walk tests or quality-of-life assessments could be discerned between the two therapies.

Discussion

Before scrutinizing the human clinical trials involving ET-antagonists, one should re-examine how ET functions in the body. Clinical agents developed for the ET arena in the past few years have focused mainly on ET-A receptor antagonism, but some agents have been nonselective. Whether it is best to antagonize the ET-A receptor, the ET-B receptor, or both is unknown. Although the ET-B receptor is associated with vasodilation, it also has been linked to aldosterone secretion in heart failure [57]. The lack of fundamental knowledge of these receptor subtypes can undermine assumptions of how specific ET receptor antagonists work. Therefore, judging a therapy as a failure mandates a closer inspection of how these receptor types might interact with one another in pathologic situations.

In relation to the post–myocardial infarction animal model experiments, the question of "therapeutic timing" is vital. The timing of administration of an ET antagonist likely is pivotal in determining positive clinical outcomes. Although many post–myocardial infarction animal models did well in relation to hemodynamic and clinical parameters, some had negative outcomes from therapy instituted early in the disease process. ET, despite having potential long-term deleterious effects on the failing heart, may help the acutely injured heart repair itself through fibroblast proliferation and tissue stability [32]. Thus timing as well as dosage may be critical when using these agents to treat post–myocardial infarction–induced heart failure.

Examining the human heart failure clinical trials, the quandary of how receptor-subtype antagonism is mediated is repeated; selective agents have not conferred significant benefits over placebo in several different clinical endpoints. The weak positive dose-related trend seen with the higher doses in the EARTH trial presents a muddled picture: with higher doses, are ET-A receptor antagonists engaged in some overlap with the ET-B receptor? Or at higher doses, is the ET-A receptor site blockaded more thoroughly? Post hoc analysis of the RITZ-5 trial revealed that patients receiving the higher dose of tezosentan had worse outcomes than patients who received placebo; patients who received the lower dose had improved outcomes compared with placebo [55]. As a nonselective agent, tezosentan is intrinsically different in function and composition than darusentan; thus, assuming that nonselective ET-receptor blockade at a low dose would be more beneficial than selective antagonism at higher doses would be inappropriate, especially given the failure of bosentan to establish this premise in the ENABLE study. Finally, blockade of ET-B receptors may have a deleterious effect on renal salt and water handling. This may explain the increased incidence of worsening heart failure seen in some trials (eg, REACH, ENABLE, ENCORE).

Summary

The number of therapeutic agents available to physicians treating patients who have heart failure seems to be expanding daily. The emphasis on receptor sites and hormonal interactions involved in the pathogenesis of heart failure results in continuous development in this area, as evidenced by the development of NEP inhibitors and ET antagonists. Unfortunately, these therapies have fallen short of their intended goal of effectively disrupting the neurohormonal cascade of heart failure. Before banishing these agents to the nether regions of the pharmaceutical spectrum, however, one should take into account the base-line knowledge, or lack thereof, of how these medications function. Is the breadth of their cellular interactions and underlying mechanisms known? Are these agents truly limited in their scope to treat heart failure because of a lack of positive results in the clinical trials? It would behoove clinicians and researchers to investigate thoroughly the basic workings of these medica-tions because they may offer clues or further insight that could aid the development of alterna-tive remedies. Otherwise, the future will bring repetition of the same labored steps with fruitless trials and another new class of supposed "wonder drugs."

References

[1] The CONSENSUS Trial Study Group. Effects of enalapril on mortality in severe congestive heart fail-ure. Results of the Cooperative North Scandinavian Enalapril Survival Study (CONSENSUS). N Engl J Med 1987;316(23):1429–35.

[2] Packer M, Bristow MR, Cohn JN, et al. The effect of carvedilol on morbidity and mortality in patients with chronic heart failure. US Carvedilol Heart Fail-ure Study Group. N Engl J Med 1996;334(21): 1349–55.

[3] Pitt B, Zannad F, Remme WJ, et al. The effect of spi-ronolactone on morbidity and mortality in patients with severe heart failure. N Engl J Med 1999;341: 709–17.

[4] Cohn JN, Tognoni G. A randomized trial of the an-giotensin-receptor blocker valsartan in chronic heart failure. N Engl J Med 2001;345:1667–75.

[5] Margulies KB, Barclay PL, Burnett JC Jr. The role of neutral endopeptidase in dogs with evolving con-gestive heart failure. Circulation 1995;91:2036–42.

[6] Graf K, Koehne P, Grafe M, et al. Regulation and differential expression of neutral endopeptidase 24. 11 in human endothelial cells. Hypertension 1995; 26:230–5.

[7] Dussaule JC, Stefanski A, Bea ML, et al. Character-ization of neutral endopeptidase in vascular smooth muscle cells of rabbit renal cortex. Am J Physiol 1993;264:F45–52.

[8] Stephenson SL, Kenny AJ. The hydrolysis of alpha-human atrial natriuretic peptide by pig kidney mi-crovillar membranes is initiated by endopeptidase 24.11. Biochem J 1987;243:183–7.

[9] Kenny AJ, Bourne A, Ingram J. Hydrolysis of hu-man and pig brain natriuretic peptides, urodilantin, C-type natriuretic peptide and some C-type receptor ligands by endopeptidase 24.11. Biochem J 1993; 291:83–8.

[10] Skidgel RA, Engelbrecht S, Johnson AR, et al. Hy-drolysis of substance P and neurotensin by convert-ing enzyme and neutral endopeptidase. Peptides 1984;5:769–76.

[11] Ogihara T, Rakugi H, Masuo K, et al. Antihyperten-sive effects of the neutral endopeptidase inhibitor SCH 42495 in essential hypertension. Am J Hyper-tens 1994;7:943–7.

[12] Singer DR, Markandu ND, Buckley MG, et al. Di-etary sodium and inhibition of neutral endopepti-dase 24.11 in essential hypertension. Hypertension 1991;18:798–804.

[13] Ando S, Rahman MA, Butler GC, et al. Comparison of candoxatril and atrial natriuretic factor in healthy men. Effects on hemodynamics, sympathetic activ-ity, heart rate variability, and endothelin. Hyperten-sion 1995;26:1160–6.

[14] Kahn JC, Patey M, Dubois-Rande JL, et al. Effect of sinorphan on plasma atrial natriuretic factor in con-gestive heart failure. Lancet 1990;335:118–9.

[15] Good JM, Peters M, Wilkins M, et al. Renal re-sponse to candoxatrilat in patients with heart failure. J Am Coll Cardiol 1995;25:1273–81.

[16] Trippodo NC, Robl JA, Asaas MM, et al. Cardio-vascular effects of the novel dual inhibitor of neutral endopeptidase and angiotensin-converting enzyme BMS-182657 in experimental hypertension and heart failure. J Pharmacol Exp Ther 1995;275: 745–52.

[17] Fournie-Zaluski MC, Coric P, Thery V, et al. Design of orally active dual inhibitors of neutral endopepti-dase and angiotensin-converting enzyme with long duration of action. J Med Chem 1996;39:2594–608.

[18] Laurent S, Boutouyric P, Azizi M, et al. Antihyper-tensive effects of fasidotril, a dual inhibitor of nepri-lysin and angiotensin-converting enzyme, in rats and humans. Hypertension 2000;35:1148–53.

[19] Wallis EJ, Ramsay LE, Hettiarachchi J. Combined inhibition of neutral endopeptidase and angioten-sin-converting enzyme by sampatrilat in essential hy-pertension. Clin Pharmacol Ther 1998;64:439–49.

[20] Trippodo NC, Robl JA, Asaad MM, et al. Effects of omapatrilat in low, normal, and high renin experi-mental hypertension. Am J Hypertens 1998;11: 363–72.

[21] Trippodo NC, Fox M, Monticello TM, et al. Vaso-peptidase inhibition with omapatrilat improves car-diac geometry and survival in cardiomyopathic hamsters more than does ACE inhibition with cap-topril. J Cardiovasc Pharmacol 1999;34:782–90.

[22] McClean DR, Ikram H, Garlick AH, et al. The clinical, cardiac, renal, arterial and neurohormonal effects of omapatrilat, a vasopeptidase inhibitor, in patients with chronic heart failure. J Am Coll Cardiol 2000;36(2):479–86.

[23] Rouleau JL, Pfeffer MA, Stewart DJ, et al. Comparison of vasopeptidase inhibitor, omapatrilat, and lisinopril on exercise tolerance and morbidity in patients with heart failure: IMPRESS randomized trial. Lancet 2000;356:615–20.

[24] Packer M, Cakiff RM, Konstam MA, et al. Comparison of omapatrilat and enalapril in patients with chronic heart failure. The Omapatrilat Versus Enalapril Randomized Trial of Utility in Reducing Events (OVERTURE). Circulation 2002;106:920–6.

[25] McClean DR, Ikram H, Mehta S, et al. Vasopeptidase inhibition with omapatrilat in chronic heart failure: acute and long-term hemodynamic and neurohumoral effects. J Am Coll Cardiol 2002;39(12): 2034–41.

[26] Messerli FH, Nussberger J. Vasopeptidase inhibition and angioedema. Lancet 2000;356:608–9.

[27] Deedwania PC. Endothelin, the bad actor in the play: a marker or mediator of cardiovascular disease. J Am Coll Cardiol 1999;33:2007–18.

[28] Yanagisawa M, Kurihara H, Kimura S, et al. A novel potent vasoconstrictor peptide produced by vascular endothelial cells. Nature 1988;332:411–5.

[29] Giaid A, Yanagisawa M, Langleben D, et al. Expression of endothelin-1 in the lungs of patients with pulmonary hypertension. N Engl J Med 1993;328: 1732–9.

[30] Ohta K, Hirata Y, Imai T, et al. Cytokine-induced release of endothelin-1 from porcine renal epithelial cell line. Biochem Biophys Res Commun 1990;169: 578–84.

[31] Kohno M, Murakawa K, Yokokawa K, et al. Production of endothelin by cultured and porcine endothelial cells; modulation by adrenaline. J Hypertens 1989;7(Suppl):S130–1.

[32] Piacentini L, Gray M, Honbo NY, et al. Endothelin-1 stimulates cardiac fibroblast proliferation through activation of protein kinase C. J Mol Cell Cardiol 2000;32:565–76.

[33] MacCarthy PA, Grocott-Mason R, Prendergast PD, et al. Contrasting inotropic effects of endogenous endothelin in the normal and failing human heart: studies with an intracoronary ETA receptor antagonist. Circulation 2000;101:142–7.

[34] Masaki T, Kimura S, Yanagisawa M, et al. Molecular and cellular mechanism of endothelin regulation: implications for vascular function. Circulation 1991; 84:1457–68.

[35] Pousset F, Isnard R, Lechat P, et al. Prognostic value of plasma endothelin-1 in patients with chronic heart failure. Eur Heart J 1997;18:254–8.

[36] Wei CM, Lerman A, Rodehoeffer RJ, et al. Endothelin in human congestive heart failure. Circulation 1994;89:1580–6.

[37] McMurray JJ, Ray SG, Abdullah I, et al. Plasma endothelin in chronic heart failure. Circulation 1992;85:1374–9.

[38] Rubin LJ, Badesch DB, Barst RJ, et al. Bosentan therapy for pulmonary arterial hypertension. N Engl J Med 2002;346:896–903.

[39] Sakai S, Miyauchi T, Kobayashi M, et al. Inhibition of myocardial endothelin pathway improves long-term survival in heart failure. Nature 1996;384: 353–5.

[40] Fraccarollo D, Hu K, Galuppo P, et al. Chronic endothelin receptor blockade attenuates progressive ventricular dilatation and improves cardiac function in rats with myocardial infarction: possible involvement of myocardial endothelin system in ventricular remodeling. Circulation 1997;96:3963–73.

[41] Hu K, Gaudron P, Schmidt TJ, et al. Aggravation of left ventricular remodeling by a novel specific endothelin ET-A antagonist EMD94246 in rats with myocardial infarction. J Cardiovasc Pharmacol 1998;32:505–8.

[42] Nguyen QT, Cernacek P, Sirois MG, et al. Long-term effects of non-selective endothelin A and B receptor antagonism in post-infarction rat: importance of timing. Circulation 2001;104:2075–81.

[43] Clozel M, Qiu C, Qiu CS, et al. Short-term endothelin receptor blockade with tezosentan has both immediate and long-term beneficial effects in rats with myocardial infarction. J Am Coll Cardiol 2002;39:142–7.

[44] Bauersachs J, Fraccarollo D, Galuppo P, et al. Endothelin receptor blockade improves endothelial vasomotor dysfunction in heart failure. Cardiovasc Res 2000;47:142–9.

[45] Saad D, Mukherjee R, Thomas P, et al. The effects of endothelin-A receptor blockade during the progression of pacing-induced congestive heart failure. J Am Coll Cardiol 1998;32:1779–86.

[46] Teerlink J, Löffler BM, Hess P, et al. Role of endothelin in the maintenance of blood pressure in conscious rats with chronic heart failure. Circulation 1994;90:2510–8.

[47] Torre-Amione G, Young JB, Durnad JB, et al. Hemodynamic effects of tezosentan, an intravenous dual endothelin receptor antagonist, in patients with class III to IV congestive heart failure. Circulation 2001;103:973–80.

[48] Berger R, Stanek B, Hulsmann M, et al. Effects of ET-A receptor blockade on endothelial function in patients with chronic heart failure. Circulation 2001;103:981–6.

[49] Mylona P, Cleland JG. Update of REACH-1 and MERIT-HF clinical trials in heart failure: Cardio. net Editorial Team. Eur J Heart Fail 1999;1: 197–200.

[50] Kalra PR, Moon JC, Coats AJ. Do results of the ENABLE study spell the end for non-selective endothelin antagonism in heart failure? Int J Cardiol 2002;85:195–7.

[51] Luscher TF, Enseleit F, Pacher R, et al. Hemody-namic and neurohormonal effects of selective endo-thelin A (ET-A) receptor blockade in chronic heart failure: the Heart Failure ET-A Receptor Blockade Trial (HEAT). Circulation 2002;106:2666–72.

[52] Louis A, Cleland JG, Crabbe S, et al. Clinical trials up-date: CAPRICORN, COPERNICUS, MIRACLE, STAF, RITZ-2, RECOVER, and RENAISSANCE and cachexia and cholesterol in heart failure: high-lights of the Scientific Sessions of the American College of Cardiology, 2001. Eur J Heart Fail 2001;3:381–7.

[53] Coletta AP, Cleland JG. Clinical trials update. High-lights of the scientific sessions of the XXIII Congress of the European Society of Cardiology: WARIS II, ESCAMI, PAFAC, RITZ-1, and TIME. Eur J Heart Fail 2001;3:747–50.

[54] O'Connor CM, Gattis WA, Adams KF, et al. Tezo-sentan in patients with acute heart failure and acute

coronary syndromes: results of the Randomized In-travenous Tezosentan Study (RITZ-4). J Am Coll Cardiol 2003;41:1452–7.

[55] Kaluski E, Kobrin I, Zimlichman R, et al. RITZ-5: Randomized Intravenous Tezosentan for the treat-ment of pulmonary edema: a prospective, multicen-ter, double-blind, placebo-controlled study. J Am Coll Cardiol 2003;41:204–10.

[56] Anand I, McMurray J, Cohn JN, et al. Long term ef-fects of darusentan on left-ventricular remodeling and clinical outcomes in the ET-A Receptor Antag-onist Trial in Heart Failure (EARTH): randomized, double-blind, placebo-controlled trial. Lancet 2004; 364:347–54.

[57] Wada A, Tsutamoto T, Fukai D, et al. Comparison of the effects of selective endothelin ET-A and ET-B receptor antagonists in congestive heart failure. J Am Coll Cardiol 1997;30:1385–92.

ELSEVIER
SAUNDERS

CARDIOLOGY
CLINICS

Cardiol Clin 26 (2008) 49–58

Anticoagulants, Antiplatelets, and Statins in Heart Failure

Dimitrios Farmakis, MD, PhD[a],
Gerasimos Filippatos, MD, PhD, FESC[a],
Mitja Lainscak, MD, PhD, FESC[b],
John T. Parissis, MD, PhD, FESC[a],
Stefan D. Anker, MD, PhD, FESC[c,d],*,
Dimitrios T. Kremastinos, MD, PhD, FESC[a]

[a]University of Athens Medical School, Attikon University Hospital, Athens, Greece
[b]The University Clinic of Respiratory and Allergic Diseases Golnik, Golnik, Slovenia
[c]Charité Campus Virchow-Klinikum, Berlin, Germany
[d]National Heart and Lung Institute, Imperial College, London, UK

Heart failure is the end-stage condition of practically every form of heart disease as well as a disease of the elderly. The already enormous socioeconomic burden related to heart failure continues to grow as the general population becomes older, cardiac diseases are managed more effectively, and life-saving therapies prolong the survival of patients already in heart failure.

Heart failure represents an extremely heterogeneous group of patients, characterized by frequent and significant comorbid conditions as well as by complications arising from a variety of heart failure–related pathogenetic mechanisms. Thus, besides the currently established life-saving therapies that are proved to ameliorate substantially patients' prognosis and survival, such as beta-blocking agents, angiotensin-converting enzyme inhibitors, and aldosterone antagonists [1–3], a number of additional medication classes have attracted the attention during the past years.

Among them, antiplatelet (APT) and anticoagulant (AC) agents and statins hold a central role. This article outlines the current knowledge regarding the use of these three drug classes in patients who have heart failure.

Antiplatelet and anticoagulant agents

The currently available guidelines for the treatment of patients who have heart failure restrict the administration of APT and AC agents only to patients who have specific comorbidities, including coronary artery disease, atrial fibrillation, a history of thromboembolic events, and left ventricular mural thrombus. The rationale for extending the application of APT or AC therapy beyond these very specific patient subgroups to the vast majority of patients who have heart failure relies, on one hand, on the occurrence of thromboembolic complications and, on the other, on the pathophysiology of the disease itself.

Heart failure is followed by an increased incidence of thromboembolic events, such as cerebrovascular accidents or venous thrombosis. This incidence is estimated to be 2%, versus only 0.5% in the general population, and may reach even 4% or 5% in patients who have severe heart

* Corresponding author. Division of Applied Cachexia Research, Department of Cardiology, Charité Campus Virchow-Klinikum, Augustenburger Platz 1, D-13353 Berlin, Germany.
E-mail address: s.anker@cachexia.de (S.D. Anker).

failure [4]. At the same time, thromboembolism is probably an underestimated cause of death in heart failure. For example, although sudden death is believed to be arrhythmogenic, autopsy data in 171 patients from the Assessment of Treatment with Lisinopril and Survival trial showed that an acute coronary event may have occurred in a significant number of patients who die suddenly, even in the absence of a history of coronary artery disease [5]. The same finding applies to death related to myocardial failure [5] On the other hand, heart failure is practically a hypercoagulable state, because it is followed by intracardiac and peripheral blood flow deceleration, endothelial dysfunction, abnormalities of hemostasis, and platelet activation [6,7].

The evidence supporting the use of APT or AC in heart failure is still limited, however, and the few randomized clinical trials have been small or underpowered. More specifically, the Warfarin/ Aspirin Study in Heart Failure study [8] randomly assigned 279 patients who had heart failure and left ventricular systolic dysfunction to one of three arms (no antithrombotic therapy; aspirin (300 mg/d); or warfarin with a target International Normalized Ratio of 2.5) and followed them for a mean of 27 months. No differences were noted among the three groups regarding the primary end points of death, nonfatal myocardial infarction, or nonfatal stroke (Fig. 1). Moreover, there was a trend toward worse outcome and a significantly increased hospitalization rate for cardiovascular reasons in patients assigned to the aspirin group (Fig. 2). The Warfarin and Antiplatelet Therapy in Heart Failure trial randomly assigned a much larger patient population of 1587 patients who had symptomatic heart failure (left ventricular ejection fraction $\leq$ 35%) and sinus rhythm to warfarin (with a target International Normalized Ratio 2.5–3.0) or antiplatelet therapy with either aspirin (162 mg/d) or clopidogrel (75 mg/d) [9]. The study was terminated earlier than expected and therefore was underpowered. No significant differences were noted in the incidence of death, nonfatal myocardial infarction, or nonfatal stroke between AC and APT therapy, whereas aspirin, once again, was correlated with a higher hospitalization rate [10]. Moreover, in the Heart Failure Long-Term Antithrombotic study, a multicenter, randomized, double-blind, placebo-controlled trial that included 197 patients who had heart failure, subjects who had ischemic heart disease were assigned randomly to either aspirin (325 mg/d) or warfarin, whereas those who had dilated cardiomyopathy were assigned randomly to either warfarin or placebo [11]. The incidence of embolic or of myocardial infarction, hospitalization, heart failure exacerbation, death, or hemorrhage did not differ significantly between the treatment arms.

In contrast to randomized trials, retrospective analyses of large cohorts of patients who have heart failure have provided important insights regarding the use of APT or AC agents in heart

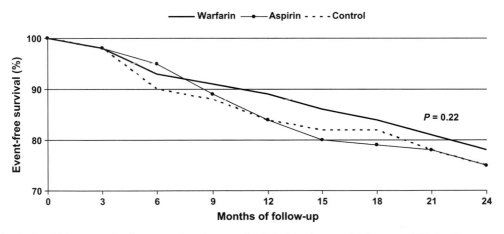

Fig. 1. Kaplan-Meier curves for the composite primary end point of death or nonfatal myocardial infarction or nonfatal stroke in the Warfarin/Aspirin Study in Heart Failure (WASH) trial (n = 279). (*Data from* Cleland JGF, Findlay I, Jafri S, et al. The Warfarin/Aspirin Study in Heart Failure (WASH): a randomized trial comparing antithrombotic strategies for patients with heart failure. Am Heart J 2004;148:157–64.)

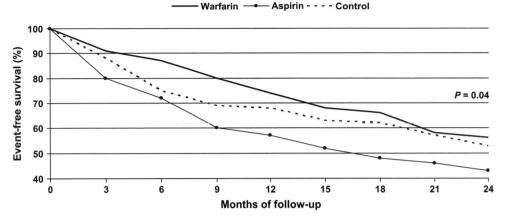

Fig. 2. Kaplan-Meier curves for the time to first hospitalization for any reason in the Warfarin/Aspirin Study in Heart Failure (WASH) trial (n = 279). (*Data from* Cleland JGF, Findlay I, Jafri S, et al. The Warfarin/Aspirin Study in Heart Failure (WASH): a randomized trial comparing antithrombotic strategies for patients with heart failure. Am Heart J 2004;148:157–64.)

failure. In a retrospective analysis of 6797 patients participating in the Studies of Left Ventricular Dysfunction who had moderate to severe left ventricular systolic dysfunction, APT and AC therapy were associated independently with a reduction in the risk of sudden coronary death of 24% and 32%, respectively [12]. In the Survival and Ventricular Enlargement trial [13], which included 2231 patients who had postmyocardial infarction left ventricular systolic dysfunction, warfarin and aspirin therapy were associated with a 81% and 56% reduction of the risk for stroke, respectively. Furthermore, a subanalysis of the Cooperative North Scandinavian Enalapril Survival Study of 253 patients who had severe congestive heart failure [4] showed that warfarin therapy was associated with a 40% reduction in mortality. Investigators in the Second Perspective Randomised Study of Ibopamine on Mortality and Efficacy performed a post hoc analysis on the effects of APT or AC therapy on mortality in 427 patients who had advanced heart failure and were followed for 3.4 years [10]. Mortality, although better in patients receiving either form of antithrombotic therapy, did not differ significantly between the patients receiving APT and those not receiving APT (41% versus 52%) or between the patients receiving AC and those not receiving AC (48% versus 55%). After adjustments for known prognostic factors, however, the use of either APT or AC was related to a better prognosis. In line with the aforementioned trials, the Epidémiologie de l'Insuffisance Cardiaque Avancée en Lorraine (EPICAL) study followed 417 patients who had severe heart failure (New York Heart Association class III or IV; left ventricular ejection fraction ≤ 30%) for an average of 5 years and showed that both AC and aspirin were associated with better survival [14]. The Veterans Affairs Vasodilator-Heart Failure Trials, in contrast, showed that the incidence of thromboembolic events was not reduced in patients who had heart failure treated with warfarin [15]. Finally, in a recently published observational study of 7352 patients discharged from 103 Canadian hospitals with the diagnosis of heart failure, aspirin use did not affect either 1-year outcome (in terms of mortality and rates of readmission for heart failure decompensation) or the beneficial effects of angiotensin-converting enzyme inhibitors in these patients [16].

The observed differences in outcomes among these trials may arise, in part, from differences in the study populations, especially in the severity of heart failure and the frequency of important comorbidities such as atrial fibrillation.

The use of antithrombotic therapy in patients who have heart failure is strongly related to the cause of heat failure. Ischemic heart disease usually is treated with APT agents [17], whereas atrial fibrillation, which is more frequent in patients who have acute heart failure, is treated with AC agents [18]. Although no prospective data support the use of antithrombotics, the clinical practice is largely different. According to the data from a large, community-based cohort (n = 7352) aspirin was used in 42% of patients, and it was not associated with an increase in the rates of mortality or of readmission for heart failure, nor did it attenuate the benefits of angiotensin-converting enzyme inhibitors [16]. Moreover, in the large, multinational EuroHeart Failure survey (n = 11,016), antithrombotics (78%) and aspirin (29%) were prescribed frequently [19]. The odds for receiving antithrombotic treatment were increased by supraventricular arrhythmia (odds ratio [OR], 2.96; 95% confidence interval [CI], 2.51–3.50) and ischemic heart disease (OR, 2.86; 95% CI, 2.41–3.39). Patients who had ischemic heart disease, in particular, had a higher chance of being treated with aspirin (OR, 5.67; 95% CI, 4.78–6.72). In a subgroup of patients who had left ventricular systolic dysfunction (n = 3658), the proportions of patients treated with aspirin or warfarin were 54% and 26%, respectively [20]. Whether this approach is beneficial for the patients is still controversial. The results of the ongoing randomized, double-blind Warfarin Versus Aspirin in Reduced Cardiac Ejection Fraction trial (Table 1), which plans to allocate

2860 patients (with a left ventricular ejection fraction ≤ 35% and without atrial fibrillation or mechanical valve prosthesis) randomly to either warfarin or aspirin, should help guide the selection of optimal antithrombotic therapy for patients who have left ventricular systolic dysfunction [21].

Statins

The introduction of 3-hydroxy-3-methylglutaryl-coenzyme A reductase inhibitors or statins in clinical practice has changed cardiovascular pharmacology dramatically with respect to the primary and secondary prevention of the clinical consequences of atherosclerosis [22–24]. In addition to their lipid-lowering effect, statins have been shown to have some additional pleiotropic properties that may allow their indications to be expanded to a broader spectrum of diseases, possibly including heart failure [25]. Indeed, there is evidence that the use of statins may be beneficial in both ischemic and nonischemic heart failure, in patients with systolic and diastolic dysfunction, and that those beneficial effects relate to prognosis and

Table 1
Ongoing or recently published clinical trials of the use of antithrombotic agents or statins in patients who have heart failure

Trial	Number of Patients and Patient Characteristics	Intervention	Primary End Point
WARCEF	2860 patients NYHA class I-IV No mechanical heart valves or atrial fibrillation LVEF ≤35%	Warfarin (INR 2.5–3) versus Aspirin (325 mg/d)	Death or stroke (ischemic or hemorrhagic)
GISSI-HF	7000 patients NYHA class II-IV Clinical evidence of heart failure of any cause according to European Society of Cardiology guidelines In case of LVEF >40%, at least one hospital admission for congestive heart failure in last 12 months required	n-3 polyunsaturated fatty acids versus placebo Patients with no clear indication or contraindication to cholesterol-lowering therapy will be randomly assigned further to rosuvastatin (10 mg/d) versus placebo	All-cause mortality or cardiovascular hospitalization
CORONA	5016 patients aged ≥60 years, NYHA class II-IV Heart failure of ischemic origin LVEF ≤40% (NYHA class III & IV) LVEF ≤35% (NYHA class II)	Rosuvastatin (10 mg/d) versus placebo	Cardiovascular death or nonfatal myocardial infarction or nonfatal stroke

Abbreviations: CORONA, Controlled Rosuvastatin Multinational Study in Heart Failure; GISSI, Gruppo Italiano per lo Studio della Sopravvivenza nell'Infarto Miocardico; INR, international normalized ratio; LVEF, left ventricular ejection fraction; NYHA, New York Heart Association; WARCEF, Warfarin Versus Aspirin in Reduced Cardiac Ejection Function.

mortality as well as to functional and exercise capacity and quality of life [25]. Moreover, statins also have been shown to prevent the development of heart failure following an acute coronary event [26].

In the Scandinavian Simvastatin Survival Study, in which 4444 patients who had known coronary heart disease but not heart failure were assigned randomly to simvastatin or placebo, simvastatin significantly reduced the occurrence of heart failure over a follow-up period of 5 years (8.3% in the simvastatin arm, versus 10.3% in the placebo arm) [27]. Similarly, in the Pravastatin or Atorvastatin Evaluation and Infection Trial–Thrombolysis In Myocardial Infarction 22 study, which randomly assigned 4162 patients who had suffered an acute coronary syndrome to intensive (atorvastatin, 80 mg/d) or conservative (pravastatin, 40 mg/d) statin therapy and followed them for 2 years, intensive statin therapy reduced the risk of hospitalization for heart failure (1.6% versus 3.1%), independently of a recurrent myocardial infarction or a prior history of heart failure [28]. Furthermore, a meta-analysis of trials enrolling a total of 27,546 patients confirmed this finding, with a 27% reduction in the risk of hospitalization for heart failure following intensive statin therapy [28].

Go and colleagues [29], after having studied a large cohort of 24,598 patients who had heart failure and no prior statin therapy, concluded that statin use was associated with a lower risk of all-cause mortality (14.5 per 100 person-years with statin therapy, versus 25.3 per 100 person-years without statin therapy) and lower risk of hospitalization for heart failure (21.9 per 100 person-years with statin therapy, versus 31.1 per 100 person-years without statin therapy), both in patients who had known coronary artery disease and in those who did not. Similarly, Foody and colleagues [30] analyzed an even larger cohort of 54,960 elderly patients (aged 65 years or older) hospitalized because of heart failure and showed that therapy with statins on discharge (16.7% of patients) was associated with a significantly lower mortality at 1 and 3 years after discharge. In another retrospective analysis of a population-based cohort of 28,828 elderly patients (aged 66–85 years) in Canada, who had newly diagnosed heart failure, followed for 7 years, statin therapy was associated with a significantly lower occurrence of the composite end point of death from all causes, nonfatal acute myocardial infarction, and nonfatal stroke (13.6 per 100 person-years in statin recipients, versus 21.8 per 100 person-years in those who did not receive statins). This

finding resulted from the reduction in all-cause mortality; no significant reduction in subsequent myocardial infarction was observed [31].

In a retrospective, nonrandomized analysis of the Optimal Therapy in Myocardial with the Angiotensin II Antagonist Losartan trial, which evaluated the effect of early-onset statin and beta-blocker therapy in 5477 patients who had heart failure following myocardial infarction, each of the two modalities alone was associated with significantly reduced all-cause mortality (26.1% risk reduction for statins, 30.6% for beta-blockers), and the beneficial effects of their combination were additive (48.3% risk reduction) [32]. Furthermore, Anker and colleagues [33] analyzed two cohorts of patients who had heart failure of ischemic and nonischemic origin: 3132 patients enrolled in the Evaluation of Losartan in the Elderly II study and another 2068 patients pooled from databases of five tertiary referral centers. One third of those patients were receiving statin therapy, which was independently associated with lower portability rates in both cohorts (adjusted hazard ratios, 0.66 and 0.58, respectively) and in patients who had heart failure of ischemic and nonischemic origin (Fig. 3). Similarly, in a cohort of 551 patients who had systolic heart failure (left ventricular ejection fraction ≤ 40%), 45% of whom had a history of coronary artery disease and another 45% of whom were receiving statin therapy, Horwich and colleagues [34] showed that statin therapy was independently associated with longer survival without the need of heart transplantation at 1 year, in both the ischemic and in the nonischemic subgroups (91% versus 72% and 81% versus 63%, respectively). Moreover, the aforementioned EPICAL study, which followed 417 patients who had severe heart failure for 5 years, also showed that lipid-lowering therapy was associated with better survival [14].

In the recently published Treating to New Targets study, 10,001 patients who had known coronary artery disease (7.8% of whom had a history of heart failure) were assigned randomly to intensive versus conservative atorvastatin therapy (80 versus 10 mg/d) and were followed for 5 years [35]. The incidence of hospitalization for heart failure was significantly lower in the intensive atorvastatin arm (2.4% versus 3.3%), and this effect was observed mainly in the subgroup of patients who had a prior history of heart failure (10.6% versus 17.3% hospitalization rates). Moreover, recently published data from the Beta-Blocker Evaluation of Survival Trial of 1024 patients who had moderate to severe heart

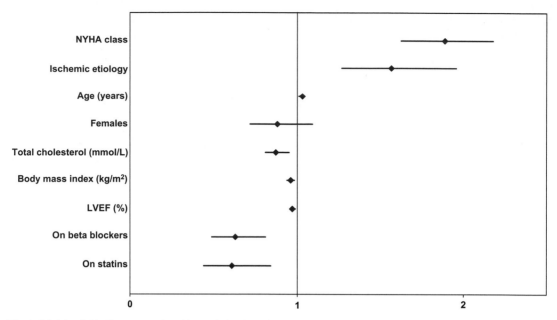

Fig. 3. Multivariable Cox proportional hazards model (with 95% confidence intervals) of factors affecting survival in the Evaluation of Losartan in the Elderly III study (n = 3082). LVEF, left ventricular ejection fraction; NYHA, New York heart Association. (*Data from* Anker SD, Clark AL, Winkler R, et al. Statin use and survival in patients with chronic heart failure—results from two observational studies with 5200 patients. Int J Cardiol 2006;112:234–42.)

failure secondary to nonischemic dilated cardiomyopathy (New York Heart Association functional class III or IV; left ventricular ejection fraction ≤ 35%) showed that statin use was independently associated with reduction of both all-cause and cardiovascular mortality [36].

Finally, regarding diastolic heart failure, Fukuta and colleagues [37] studied 137 patients with heart failure and preserved left ventricular ejection fraction (≥ 50%). During a mean follow-up of 21 months, statin therapy was associated with significantly lower mortality (adjusted relative risk, 0.20).

Despite these encouraging results, a very recent overview of trials of the use of statins in heart failure pointed out that the accumulated body of evidence is limited because the corresponding studies are either retrospective and observational or are small, prospective studies. Other limitations are the use of incompletely validated end points and non-uniform statin regimens [38]. The potential beneficial effects of statins are obviously incompletely explained by their lipid-reduction effect. Thus additional mechanisms probably are involved, and these mechanisms probably lie in the pleiotropic properties of these drugs.

First, statins are known to have anti-inflammatory effects, and these effects also have been observed in patients who have heart failure. Thus, Mozaffarian and colleagues [39] studied 22 patients, most of whom had nonischemic heart failure (New York Heart Association class II or III; left ventricular ejection fraction < 40%), who received atorvastatin (10 mg/d) in a randomized and cross-over manner. Statin treatment reduced the serum levels of soluble tumor necrosis factor (TNF) receptor-1 by 8%, of C-reactive protein by 37%, and of endothelin-1 by 17%. Similarly, Tousoulis and colleagues [40] showed that atorvastatin (10 mg/d) reduced serum concentration of interleukin-6 and TNF-α after 4 weeks in a group of 38 patients who had ischemic cardiomyopathy and were assigned randomly to atorvastatin, atorvastatin plus vitamin E, or neither of the two agents. In this interesting study, the investigators also observed a significant reduction in the serum levels of vascular cell adhesion molecule, as well as an improvement in endothelial function, as evaluated by the forearm vasodilatory response to reactive hyperemia, following the 4-week, low-dose atorvastatin therapy [40]. In another study, Tousoulis and colleagues [41] showed that the same statin regimen modified the expression of several components of the thrombosis-fibrinolysis system in a group of 35 patients who had heart failure assigned randomly to atorvastatin or placebo. More specifically, they showed a significant decline in plasma concentrations of antithrombin III, protein C, factor V, tissue plasminogen activator factor, and plasminogen activator inhibitor factor after 4 weeks of treatment; no effect was observed in the levels of von Willebrand's factor, factor VII, and protein S [41]. Thus, besides their anti-inflammatory effects, statins also may improve endothelial function and confer an antithrombotic effect in patients who have heart failure. Moreover, Landmesser and colleagues [42] studied the effects of atorvastatin after myocardial infarction in an experimental model of wild-type and endothelial nitric oxide synthase–knockout mice. Four weeks of atorvastatin therapy resulted in a significant amelioration of endothelium-dependent, nitric oxide–mediated vasodilatation, mobilization of endothelial progenitor cells, neovascularization of peri-infarct area, and survival, as well as in a significant attenuation of left ventricular dysfunction and myocardial interstitial fibrosis (in wild-type mice only) [42]. In dogs with microembolization-induced heart failure, 3-month therapy with rosuvastatin prevented progressive cardiac remodeling. This effect may be derived partly from decreased TNF-α expression and enhanced mobilization of bone marrow–derived stem cells [43]. In addition, statins seem to attenuate the increased sympathetic tone, which characterizes neurohormonal activation in heart failure. In an experimental heart failure model in rabbits, high-dose simvastatin therapy normalized renal sympathetic nerve activity; statins also may improve heart rate variability [25]. The pleiotropic effects of statins on the failing myocardium are summarized in Box 1.

On the other hand, there are reports that statins may be harmful in patients who have heart failure. Low total cholesterol levels have been associated with worse outcome in terms of survival, as shown in a cohort of 1134 patients who had advanced heart failure [44]. Thus, in theory, statins may affect prognosis by lowering cholesterol levels in patients who have heart failure. According to the endotoxin-lipoprotein hypothesis [45], lipoproteins are beneficial because they bind lipopolysaccharides, which act as endotoxins, thereby leading to inflammatory activation, a well-established pathogenetic mechanism of heart failure development and progression. Thus, a lower lipoprotein concentration following total cholesterol reduction is potentially harmful in patients who have heart failure. It is not clear, however, whether the low cholesterol levels may simply be an epiphenomenon of severe heart failure, which by itself bears a worse prognosis [25].

Finally, there also is some conflicting evidence regarding the interference of statin therapy in coenzyme Q10 availability and function and the role of the latter in patients who have heart failure and in those who do not. Coenzyme Q10, or ubiquinone, is a lipophilic substituted benzoquinone that serves as a redox component of the mitochondrial respiratory chain as well as a component of extramitochondrial electron transport chains and is a powerful antioxidant and membrane stabilizer [46]. Coenzyme Q10 is reduced in patients who have heart failure [26]. A systematic literature survey on randomized, controlled trials of Q10 in chronic heart failure showed that Q10 improved left ventricular ejection fraction and increased cardiac output, hence improving systolic function in those patients [47].

The effects of statins on Q10 levels are not yet clarified. It has been shown that simvastatin therapy resulted in a significant reduction of plasma Q10 levels in a group of 20 hyperlipidemic patients [48]. In another study of 20 healthy individuals treated with either pravastatin or atorvastatin for 4 weeks in a randomized, crossover manner, however, statins did not induce a reduction of circulating Q10 [49]. The issue became even more complicated when Strey and colleagues [50] showed that statin therapy improved endothelial function in parallel with a reduction of Q10 in patients who had heart failure. More specifically, in a group of 24 patients who had heart failure (New York Heart Association class II or III; left ventricular ejection fraction < 40%) who received atorvastatin and placebo for 6 weeks each in a randomized, crossover fashion, atorvastatin improved endothelium-dependent vasodilatation, and this improvement correlated with

---

Box 1. Pleiotropic effects of statins on the failing heart

1. Reduced cytokine expression
2. Reduced expression of angiotensin II receptor I
3. Decreased cardiac sympathetic nerve activity
4. Improved coronary endothelial function
5. Increased mobilization of progenitor endothelial cells and neo-angiogenesis
6. Antifibrotic properties

a concomitant reduction of Q10 levels [50]. These findings and the aforementioned conflicting pieces of evidence suggest that much further research is needed before statins become a recognized treatment modality in patients who have heart failure without any of the already established indications for this class of drugs exists.

The role of statin therapy in patients with heart failure is addressed by a recently presented large-scale, randomized trial and another one on-going trial [51]. The Controlled rosuvastatin multinational study in heart failure (CORONA) randomized study 5011 older patients (aged ≥ 60 years) with moderate to severe systolic heart failure due to coronary artery disease to receive either rosuvastatin 10 mg/d or placebo [52]. After a 2.7 years of follow-up, no difference was noted between the two study arms in the primary end-point of cardiovascular death, non-fatal myocardial infarction and non-fatal stroke. However, a trend towards a lower incidence of non-fatal infarction of non-fatal stroke ($P = 0.05$), as well as a significant reduction of all cause, cardiovascular and heart failure hospitalization in the rosuvastatin arm. The on-going randomized clinical trial on statin therapy in heart failure, the GISSI-HF study, has been designed to randomize 7000 patients with heart failure of any etiology, left ventricular ejection fractions of 40% or lower and NYHA class II to IV symptoms to either n-3 polyunsaturated fatty acids or placebo and subsequently to rosuvastatin 10 mg/d or placebo [53].

References

[1] Colucci WS, Packer M, Bristow MR, et al. Carvedilol inhibits clinical progression in patients with mild symptoms of heart failure. US Carvedilol Heart Failure Study Group. Circulation 1996;94:2800–6.
[2] The SOLVD Investigators. Effect of enalapril on survival in patients with reduced left ventricular ejection fractions and congestive heart failure. N Engl J Med 1991;325:293–302.
[3] Pitt B, Remme W, Zannad F, et al, Eplerenone Post-Acute Myocardial Infarction Heart Failure Efficacy and Survival Study Investigators. Eplerenone, a selective aldosterone blocker, in patients with left ventricular dysfunction after myocardial infarction. N Engl J Med 2003;348:1309–21.
[4] The CONSENSUS Trial Study Group. Effects of enalapril on mortality in severe congestive heart failure. Results of the Cooperative North Scandinavian Enalapril Survival Study (CONSENSUS). N Engl J Med 1987;316:1429–35.
[5] Uretsky BF, Thygesen K, Armstrong PW, et al. Acute coronary findings at autopsy in heart failure

patients with sudden death: results from the Assessment of Treatment with Lisinopril and Survival (ATLAS) trial. Circulation 2000;102:611–6.
[6] Lip GY, Gibbs CR. Does heart failure confer a hypercoagulable state? Virchow's triad revisited. J Am Coll Cardiol 1999;33:1424–6.
[7] Dotsenko O, Kakkar VV. Antithrombotic therapy in patients with chronic heart failure: rationale, clinical evidence and practical implications. J Thromb Haemost 2007;5:224–31.
[8] Cleland JGF, Findlay I, Jafri S, et al. The Warfarin/Aspirin Study in Heart Failure (WASH): a randomized trial comparing antithrombotic strategies for patients with heart failure. Am Heart J 2004;148:157–64.
[9] Massie BM, Krol WF, Ammon SE, et al. The Warfarin and Antiplatelet Therapy in Heart Failure trial (WATCH): rationale, design, and baseline patient characteristics. J Card Fail 2004;10:101–12.
[10] de Boer RA, Hillege HL, Tjeerdsma G, et al. Both antiplatelet and anticoagulant therapy may favorably affect outcome in patients with advanced heart failure. A retrospective analysis of the PRIME-II trial. Thromb Res 2005;116:279–85.
[11] Cokkinos DV, Haralabopoulos GC, Kostis JB, et al. HELAS investigators. Efficacy of antithrombotic therapy in chronic heart failure: the HELAS study. Eur J Heart Fail 2006;8:428–32.
[12] Dries DL, Domanski MJ, Waclawiw MA, et al. Effect of antithrombotic therapy on risk of sudden coronary death in patients with congestive heart failure. Am J Cardiol 1997;79:909–13.
[13] Pfeffer MA, Braunwald E, Moye LA, et al. Effect of captopril on mortality and morbidity in patients with left ventricular dysfunction after myocardial infarction. Results of the survival and ventricular enlargement trial. The SAVE Investigators. N Engl J Med 1992;327:669–77.
[14] Echemann M, Alla F, Briancon S, et al. EPICAL Investigators Epidemiologie de l'Insuffisance Cardiaque Avancee en Lorraine. Antithrombotic therapy is associated with better survival in patients with severe heart failure and left ventricular systolic dysfunction (EPICAL study). Eur J Heart Fail 2002;4:647–54.
[15] Dunkman WB, Johnson GR, Carson PE, et al. Incidence of thromboembolic events in congestive heart failure. The V-HeFT VA Cooperative Studies Group. Circulation 1993;87:VI94–01.
[16] McAlister FA, Ghali WA, Gong Y, et al. Aspirin use and outcomes in a community-based cohort of 7352 patients discharged after first hospitalization for heart failure. Circulation 2006;113(22):2572–8.
[17] Massie BM. Aspirin use in chronic heart failure: what should we recommend to the practitioner? J Am Coll Cardiol 2005;46(6):963–6.
[18] Fuster V, Ryden LE, Cannom DS, et al. American College of Cardiology/American Heart Association, Committee for Practice Guidelines, European Society of Cardiology, European Heart Rhythm

Association; Heart Rhythm Society. ACC/AHA/ ESC 2006 guidelines for the management of patients with atrial fibrillation-executive summary: a report of the American College of Cardiology/American Heart Association Task Force on practice guidelines and the European Society of Cardiology Committee for Practice Guidelines (Writing Committee to Revise the 2001 Guidelines for the Management of Patients with Atrial Fibrillation). Eur Heart J 2006; 27(16):1979–2030.

[19] Komajda M, Follath F, Swedberg K, et al. Study Group on Diagnosis of the Working Group on Heart Failure of the European Society of Cardiology. The EuroHeart Failure Survey programme– a survey on the quality of care among patients with heart failure in Europe. Part 2: treatment. Eur Heart J 2003;24(5):464–74.

[20] Lainscak M, Cleland JG, Lenzen MJ, et al. International variations in the treatment and co-morbidity of left ventricular systolic dysfunction: data from the EuroHeart Failure Survey. Eur J Heart Fail 2007;9(3):292–9.

[21] Pullicino P, Thompson JL, Barton B, et al, WARCEF Investigators. Warfarin versus aspirin in patients with reduced cardiac ejection fraction (WARCEF): rationale, objectives, and design. J Card Fail 2006;12(1):39–46.

[22] Randomised trial of cholesterol lowering in 4444 patients with coronary heart disease: the Scandinavian Simvastatin Survival Study (4S). Lancet 1994;344: 1383–9.

[23] Shepherd J, Blauw GJ, Murphy MB, et al, PROSPER study group. Prospective study of pravastatin in the elderly at risk. Pravastatin in elderly individuals at risk of vascular disease (PROSPER): a randomised controlled trial. Lancet 2002;360: 1623–30.

[24] Sever PS, Dahlof B, Poulter NR, et al, ASCOT investigators. Prevention of coronary and stroke events with atorvastatin in hypertensive patients who have average or lower-than-average cholesterol concentrations, in the Anglo-Scandinavian cardiac outcomes trial–lipid lowering arm (ASCOT-LLA): a multicentre randomised controlled trial. Lancet 2003;361:1149–58.

[25] van der Harst P, Voors AA, van Gilst WH, et al. Statins in the treatment of chronic heart failure: biological and clinical considerations. Cardiovasc Res 2006;71:443–54.

[26] Lipinski MJ, Abbate A, Fuster V, et al. Drug insight: statins for nonischemic heart failure—evidence and potential mechanisms. Nat Clin Pract Cardiovasc Med 2007;4:196–205.

[27] Kjekshus J, Pedersen TR, Olsson AG, et al. The effects of simvastatin on the incidence of heart failure in patients with coronary heart disease. J Card Fail 1997;3:249–54.

[28] Scirica BM, Morrow DA, Cannon CP, et al, PROVE IT-TIMI 22 Investigators. Intensive statin therapy and the risk of hospitalization for heart failure after an acute coronary syndrome in the PROVE IT-TIMI 22 study. J Am Coll Cardiol 2006;47: 2326–31.

[29] Go AS, Lee WY, Yang J, et al. Statin therapy and risks for death and hospitalization in chronic heart failure. JAMA 2006;296:2105–11.

[30] Foody JM, Shah R, Galusha D, et al. Statins and mortality among elderly patients hospitalized with heart failure. Circulation 2006;113:1086 92.

[31] Ray JG, Gong Y, Sykora K, et al. Statin use and survival outcomes in elderly patients with heart failure. Arch Intern Med 2005;165:62–7.

[32] Hognestad A, Dickstein K, Myhre E, et al, OPTIMAAL Investigators. Effect of combined statin and beta-blocker treatment on one-year morbidity and mortality after acute myocardial infarction associated with heart failure. Am J Cardiol 2004;93: 603–6.

[33] Anker SD, Clark AL, Winkler R, et al. Statin use and survival in patients with chronic heart failure— results from two observational studies with 5200 patients. Int J Cardiol 2006;112:234–42.

[34] Horwich TB, MacLellan WR, Fonarow GC. Statin therapy is associated with improved survival in ischemic and non-ischemic heart failure. J Am Coll Cardiol 2004;43:642–8.

[35] Khush KK, Waters DD, Bittner V, et al. Effect of high-dose atorvastatin on hospitalizations for heart failure: subgroup analysis of the Treating to New Targets (TNT) study. Circulation 2007;115:576–83.

[36] Domanski M, Coady S, Fleg J, et al. Effect of statin therapy on survival in patients with nonischemic dilated cardiomyopathy (from the Beta-Blocker Evaluation of Survival Trial [BEST]). Am J Cardiol 2007; 99:1448–50.

[37] Fukuta H, Sane DC, Brucks S, et al. Statin therapy may be associated with lower mortality in patients with diastolic heart failure: a preliminary report. Circulation 2005;112:357–63.

[38] Martin JH, Krum H. Statins and clinical outcomes in heart failure. Clin Sci (Lond) 2007;113:119–27.

[39] Mozaffarian D, Minami E, Letterer RA, et al. The effects of atorvastatin (10 mg) on systemic inflammation in heart failure. Am J Cardiol 2005;96: 1699–704.

[40] Tousoulis D, Antoniades C, Vassiliadou C, et al. Effects of combined administration of low dose atorvastatin and vitamin E on inflammatory markers and endothelial function in patients with heart failure. Eur J Heart Fail 2005;7:1126–32.

[41] Tousoulis D, Antoniades C, Bosinakou E, et al. Effects of atorvastatin on reactive hyperaemia and the thrombosis-fibrinolysis system in patients with heart failure. Heart 2005;91:27–31.

[42] Landmesser U, Engberding N, Bahlmann FH, et al. Statin-induced improvement of endothelial progenitor cell mobilization, myocardial neovascularization, left ventricular function, and survival

after experimental myocardial infarction requires endothelial nitric oxide synthase. Circulation 2004; 110:1933–9.

[43] Zacà V, Rastogi S, Imai M, et al. Chronic monotherapy with rosuvastatin prevents progressive left ventricular dysfunction and remodeling in dogs with heart failure. J Am Coll Cardiol 2007;50:551–7.

[44] Horwich TB, Hamilton MA, Maclellan WR, et al. Low serum total cholesterol is associated with marked increase in mortality in advanced heart failure. J Card Fail 2002;8:216–24.

[45] Rauchhaus M, Coats AJ, Anker SD. The endotoxin-lipoprotein hypothesis. Lancet 2000;356:930–3.

[46] Rauchova H, Drahota Z, Lenaz G. Function of coenzyme Q in the cell: some biochemical and physiological properties. Physiol Res 1995;44:209–16.

[47] Sander S, Coleman CI, Patel AA, et al. The impact of coenzyme Q10 on systolic function in patients with chronic heart failure. J Card Fail 2006;12:464–72.

[48] Watts GF, Castelluccio C, Rice-Evans C, et al. Plasma coenzyme Q (ubiquinone) concentrations in patients treated with simvastatin. J Clin Pathol 1993;46:1055–7.

[49] Bleske BE, Willis RA, Anthony M, et al. The effect of pravastatin and atorvastatin on coenzyme Q10. Am Heart J 2001;142:E2.

[50] Strey CH, Young JM, Molyneux SL, et al. Endothelium-ameliorating effects of statin therapy and coenzyme Q10 reductions in chronic heart failure. Atherosclerosis 2005;179:201–6.

[51] Shanes JG, Minadeo KN, Moret A, et al. Statin therapy in heart failure: prognostic effects and potential mechanisms. Am Heart J 2007;154: 617–23.

[52] Kjekshus J, Apetrei E, Barrios V, et al. The CORONA Group. Rosuvastatin in Older Patients with Systolic Heart Failure. N Engl J Med 2007, (in press).

[53] Tavazzi L, Tognoni G, Franzosi MG, et al, on behalf of the GISSI-HF Investigators. Rationale and design of the GISSI heart failure trial: a large trial to assess the effects of n-3 polyunsaturated fatty acids and rosuvastatin in symptomatic congestive heart failure. Eur J Heart Fail 2004;6: 635–41.

Traditional and Novel Approaches to Management of Heart Failure: Successes and Failures

Inder S. Anand, MD, FRCP, DPhil (Oxon), FACC[a,b,*],
Viorel G. Florea, MD, PhD, ScD, FACC[a,b]

[a]Division of Cardiology, University of Minnesota Medical School, 420 Delaware Street SE,
MMC 508, Minneapolis, MN 55455, USA
[b]Heart Failure Clinic, Veterans Administration Medical Center, Cardiology 111-C, 1 Veterans Drive,
Minneapolis, MN 55417, USA

It is now generally recognized that heart failure (HF) progresses through a process of structural remodeling of the heart, to which neur.ohormonal (NH) and cytokine activation make an important contribution [1]. Several lines of evidence support the role of neurohormones in the progression of HF. Norepinephrine [2], angiotensin II [3], and cytokines [4] are directly toxic to cardiac myocytes; the degree of neurohormonal activation in HF is proportional to disease severity, increases with the progression of HF, and is related to prognosis [5]. Furthermore, changes in NH activation over time, occurring either spontaneously or in response to pharmacologic therapy, are also associated with proportional changes in subsequent mortality and morbidity [6]. These findings support the hypothesis that blocking the deleterious effects of vasoconstrictive hormones and stimulating production of vasodilator hormones would have beneficial effects. The spectacular success in reducing HF morbidity and mortality by inhibiting the sympathetic and renin-angiotensin-aldosterone systems with beta-blockers, angiotensin converting enzyme-inhibitors (ACE-I), and aldosterone receptor antagonists further underscores the importance of NH activation in the progression of HF [7–11], and raises the question as to whether an even more complete blockade of the NH system using new novel therapies would provide incremental benefit. Over the last decade the authors have been testing this hypothesis. However, recent clinical trial data evaluating strategies using novel NH blockers beyond ACE inhibition, beta-blockers, and aldosterone antagonists, have recently failed to improve the clinical outcomes of HF patients, and in some cases has even shown to be deleterious [12–16].

How do we explain the remarkable success with blockers of the adrenergic and renin-angiotensin-aldosterone system, and why have the newer novel agents had neutral or even deleterious effects on HF outcomes? In this article, the authors provide evidence that agents that have beneficial effects in HF also generally attenuate or reverse ventricular remodeling, whereas the newer novel agents that have failed to improve clinical outcomes either had no effect on remodeling or have been associated with adverse remodeling.

Blockade of the sympathetic nervous system

Beta-blockers reduce mortality in patients with New York Heart Association (NYHA) class II to IV HF by 34% to 35% [9,10,17]. These effects were associated with significant reversal of ventricular remodeling [18,19].

Excessive blockade of the sympathetic nervous system

The association between the degree of sympathetic activation and mortality [6,20] and dose-dependent favorable effects of beta-blockers on

* Corresponding author. Veterans Administration Medical Center, Cardiology 111-C, 1 Veterans Drive, Minneapolis, MN 55417.
E-mail address: anand001@umn.edu (I.S. Anand).

0733-8651/08/$ - see front matter. Published by Elsevier Inc.
doi:10.1016/j.ccl.2008.01.001

left ventricular (LV) ejection fraction and mortality [21] raised the possibility that a "more complete" adrenergic blockade might produce even greater benefit on outcomes. Moxonidine, a centrally acting α-agonist that greatly reduces circulating catecholamines [22], was used to test this hypothesis in the Moxonidine in Congestive Heart Failure trial [23]. The study had to be terminated early, with only 1,934 of the 4,533 subjects randomized because of a 38% higher mortality in the moxonidine group. Hospitalizations for HF and myocardial infarctions were also increased. The increase in mortality and morbidity was accompanied by significant decrease in plasma norepinephrine by moxonidine (−18.8%) as compared with placebo (+6.9%) [23]. It is likely that the marked sympatholytic effects of moxonidine could have produced severe myocardial depression, bradycardia, or hypotension, though this could not be documented in the subjects who died. Data on ventricular remodeling is not available from that study.

Another example of the association between marked sympatholytic effect and adverse outcomes was seen in a subgroup of patients in the Beta-blocker Evaluation of Survival trial (BEST) [24], which is the only beta-blocker HF trial that failed to demonstrate mortality benefit. This could be related to the marked sympatholytic effects of bucindolol, not seen with carvedilol or metoprolol. In BEST, subjects receiving bucindolol, who had a decrease in norepinephrine of greater than 224 pg/mL from baseline to 3 months, had a 169% increase in mortality when compared with subjects who had no significant change in norepinephrine [25].

These two examples underscore the fact that severe decrease in adrenergic support may render the body devoid of any compensatory mechanisms, resulting in adverse outcomes. Therefore, a more comprehensive blockade of the adrenergic nervous system is not a viable strategy.

Blockade of the renin-angiotensin-aldosterone system

The beneficial effects of blocking the renin-angiotensin system with ACE-I in symptomatic and asymptomatic heart failure [7,8,26] and in patients with post myocardial infarction and LV dysfunction [27–29] is also associated with attenuation of ventricular remodeling [30,31]. Would a more complete blockade of the renin-angiotensin system provide further benefit?

Effect of high-dose versus low-dose ACE-I in heart failure

Two studies have compared the effects of low- versus high-dose ACE-I in patients with moderate to severe HF. The ATLAS (Assessment of Treatment with Lisinopril And Survival) study randomly assigned 3,164 subjects with NYHA class II to IV HF and an ejection fraction less than or equal to 30% to either low doses (2.5 mg to 5.0 mg daily) or high doses (32.5 mg to 35 mg daily) of the ACE-I lisinopril for a median of 45.7 months [32]. When compared with the low-dose group, subjects in the high-dose group had a nonsignificant 8% lower risk of death ($P = .128$) but a significant 12% lower risk of death or hospitalization for any reason ($P = .002$), and 24% fewer hospitalizations for HF ($P = .002$).

The second study was much smaller and compared a very high dose of enalapril (average 42 mg plus or minus 19.3 mg per day) with usual dose (average 17.9 mg plus or minus 4.3 mg per day) and could not find any benefit of high-dose ACE-I [33]. This relative lack of beneficial effect with "excessive" blockade of ACE could be related to the phenomenon of "angiotensin II and aldosterone escape" seen with the use of ACE-I, despite complete blockade of ACE. Tang and colleagues [34] have shown that whereas high-dose enalapril (40 mg per day) caused a much greater suppression of serum ACE activity, levels of angiotensin and aldosterone remained elevated to the same extent in both the high- and low-dose ACE-I groups. Thus, high doses of ACE-I produce only minimal or no incremental benefit but are associated with more adverse side effects.

Effect of dual ACE-I and angiotensin receptor blockers in heart failure

Because physiologically active levels of angiotensin II persist despite chronic ACE inhibitor therapy [35,36], three separate studies, Val-HeFT (Valsartan Heart Failure Trial) [12], CHARM (Candesartan in Heart failure: Assessment of Reduction in Mortality and Morbidity) [37–40], and the Valsartan In Acute Myocardial Infarction [41] trials were undertaken to determine whether angiotensin receptor blockers (ARB) could further reduce morbidity and mortality in patients already receiving an ACE-I. Val-HeFT showed that the addition of valsartan to ACE-I did not reduce mortality, but caused a 28% reduction in hospitalizations for HF. However, in the 7% of subjects not receiving an ACE-I at baseline, a highly significant 41% reduction in mortality was seen [42]. The CHARM study later confirmed these findings with the use of candesartan [37–40]. Were the beneficial effects accompanied by improvement in LV structure and function? Indeed, use of valsartan in Val-HeFT was associated with improvement in LV remodeling in all subgroups of subjects except those receiving both ACE-I and beta-blockers at baseline, in whom addition of valsartan was not associated with any benefit, and this was associated with a neutral effect on remodeling [43].

Role of aldosterone receptor antagonists

Aldosterone may contribute to structural remodeling of the LV through its effects on the extracellular matrix, collagen deposition, myocardial fibrosis, and some other unique mechanisms [44–46]. Aldosterone is also important in the pathogenesis of salt and water retention in heart failure [47]. The Randomized Aldactone Evaluation Study showed a 30% reduction in mortality with spironolactone in subjects with advanced HF [11]. More recently, the Eplerenone Post-Acute Myocardial Infarction Heart Failure Efficacy and Survival study has confirmed in a postmyocardial infarction population the efficacy of an aldosterone inhibitor, in this case eplerenone, in reducing mortality in patients receiving ACE inhibitors or beta-blockers [48]. Spironolactone has also been shown to attenuate ventricular remodeling after myocardial infarction [49]. Thus, the beneficial effects of aldosterone receptor blockade on mortality are also associated with beneficial effects on LV remodeling.

Nitrates and hydralazine

Nitric oxide regulates cardiovascular processes, including myocardial hypertrophy and remodeling, as well as vascular function, inflammation, and thrombosis [50–54]. Substantial evidence exists that endothelial dysfunction and impaired bioavailability of nitric oxide occur in both ischemic and nonischemic models of HF and contribute to the pathophysiology of congestive HF [55–58]. Basal release of nitric oxide is decreased in HF [59] and the sensitivity to inhibition of nitric oxide synthase is increased [60]. Even before nitric oxide was discovered, the first Vasodilator Heart Failure Trial (V-HeFT I) [61] demonstrated the benefit of combining the nitric oxide donor isosorbide dinitrate with the antioxidant hydralazine in patients with mild-to-severe HF. The African American Heart Failure Trial (A-HeFT) confirmed the findings in V-HeFT I, even on top of ACE-I and beta blockers [62]. Once again, the mortality benefit with an isosorbide hydralazine combination was accompanied by regression of LV remodeling [61,63,64].

Role of endothelin antagonists

Like norepinephrine and angiotensin II, endothelin (ET)-1 also plays a pivotal role in cardiovascular regulation [65,66]. Plasma concentrations of ET-1 and big ET-1 are elevated in HF [67,68] and are independent predictors of mortality [69]. In advanced HF, ET_A receptors and endothelin-converting-enzyme-1 are up-regulated [70]. In a rat model of HF, ET_A-blockade improves survival [71]. Both ET_A selective (darusentan), and mixed $ET_{A/B}$ receptor antagonists (bosentan) appeared promising because single-dose administration of these agents increased cardiac output and reduced systemic and pulmonary vascular resistance in patients with severe congestive HF [72,73]. In the Research on Endothelin Antagonism in Chronic Heart Failure (REACH-1) trial [13], bosentan caused early worsening of HF but tended to improve symptoms at 6 months, suggesting a possible long-term benefit. REACH-1 was terminated prematurely because of a reversible increase in liver transaminases.

Because the nonselective $ET_{A/B}$ receptor antagonist bosentan did not show any long-term beneficial effects in HF, and because selective ET_B receptor blockade worsens hemodynamics in patients with HF [74], a selective ET_A receptor antagonist was postulated to be more effective than the mixed $ET_{A/B}$. The EndothelinA Receptor Antagonist Trial in Heart Failure investigated the chronic effects of different doses of the orally active ET_A-antagonist darusentan in 642 subjects with NYHA class II to IV HF. Over 98% of these subjects were receiving ACE-I or ARB and 80% beta-blockers. The primary endpoint was a change in LV end-systolic volume at 24 weeks, compared with baseline, measured by magnetic resonance imaging. Secondary endpoints included changes in LV mass, LV end-diastolic volume, ejection fraction, neurohormones, 6-minute walk test, quality of life, and NYHA class. Darusentan did not provide any clinical benefit, and there was no significant change in the primary endpoint of

LV end systolic volume or the other endpoints. Worsening HF was observed in 11.1% of the subjects, and 4.7% of the subjects died during the 6 month study, with no difference between groups. Darusentan had no adverse effects on neurohormones, heart rate or blood pressure [16]. Thus, the use of selective or nonselective endothelin receptor inhibitors also does not seem to add any incremental benefit in patients adequately treated with beta-blockers and ACE-I, possibly because they could not attenuate or reverse LV remodeling.

Dual angiotensin converting enzyme and neutral endopeptidase inhibition

According to the NH model of the progression of HF, blocking the deleterious effects of the vasoconstrictive hormones and stimulating the vasodilators are likely to have beneficial effects on hemodynamics, LV remodeling, and survival. Because a majority of the circulating brain natriuretic peptide (BNP) is cleared by neutral endopeptidases (NEP), the dual ACE and NEP inhibitor omapatrilat was used to test the hypothesis of blocking the renin-angiotensin system and increasing BNP. The OVERTURE (Omapatrilat Versus Enalapril Randomized Trial of Utility in Reducing Events) trial compared the effects of enalapril (20 mg per day) and omapatrilat (40 mg per day) in 5,770 subjects with NYHA class II to IV HF [14]. The primary endpoint of death and hospitalization for HF was not different in the enalapril and omapatrilat groups, but the study fulfilled the prespecified criteria of noninferiority for omapatrilat. Omapatrilat however, did reduce the combined risk of cardiovascular deaths or hospitalization by 9% ($P = .024$). Although the event rate in these high-risk subjects was high, lack of incremental benefit may have been related to significant episodes of hypotension during the period of drug up-titration. Thus, the OVERTURE trial with dual ACE and NEP inhibition is another example of how excessive use of NH inhibition may result in significant hypotension, again emphasizing that lack of attenuation of LV remodeling may be responsible for the lack of beneficial effects on outcomes.

Role of cytokine inhibition

Proinflammatory cytokines, including tumor necrosis factor (TNF)-α, interleukin (IL)-1, and IL-6, are overexpressed in HF and are involved in the progression of the disease [75]. Two approaches were used to antagonize the proinflammatory cytokine TNF-α in patients with HF-soluble TNF receptors and monoclonal antibodies.

Soluble tumor necrosis factor receptors

The first approach involved the use of etanercept (Enbrel), a genetically engineered recombinant human TNF receptor protein that binds to circulating TNF-α, and prevents TNF-α from binding to TNF receptors on target cell surface. Early preclinical studies showed that etanercept reversed the deleterious negative inotropic effects of TNF in vitro [76] and in patients with moderate to severe HF. These short-term studies in small numbers of subjects showed improvements in quality of life, 6-minute walk distance, and LV ejection fraction after 3 months treatment with etanercept [77,78].

These encouraging findings lead to the design of two multicenter clinical trials in subjects with NYHA class III to IV HF: the RENAISSANCE (Randomized Etanercept North American Strategy to Study Antagonism of Cytokines) study ($n = 900$) in the United States, and the RECOVER (Research into Etanercept Cytokine Antagonism in Ventricular Dysfunction) study ($n = 900$), in Europe and Australia. Both trials had parallel study design but differed in the doses of etanercept that were used: RENAISSANCE used doses of 25 mg twice a week and 25 mg three times a week, whereas RECOVER used doses of 25 mg once a week and 25 mg twice a week. The primary endpoint of these trials was a clinical composite. A third trial, termed Randomized Etanercept Worldwide Evaluation (RENEWAL) ($n = 1,500$) pooled the data from the RENAISSANCE (twice and three times a week dosing) and RECOVER (twice a week dosing only), and had all-cause mortality and hospitalization for heart failure as the primary endpoint. The Data Monitoring Safety Board stopped the studies early because it was felt that the studies were unlikely to show a benefit in the primary endpoints if allowed to be completed [79]. Preliminary analysis of the data showed no benefit for etanercept on the clinical composite endpoint in RENAISSANCE and RECOVER, nor a benefit for etanercept on all-cause mortality and HF hospitalizations in RENEWAL [80].

In a post hoc analysis, however, the hazard ratios for death or hospitalization for worsening

HF in subjects taking the twice a week dose of etanercept in RECOVER, was 0.87, as compared to 1.21 and 1.23 for the subjects in RENAISSANCE receiving etanercept twice a week and three times a week, respectively. These disparities in study findings were considered to be related to the different length of follow-up in the two studies. Subjects in RECOVER received etanercept for a median time of 5.7 months, whereas subjects in RENAISSANCE received etanercept for 12.7 months [4]. This suggests that the longer the exposure to the drug, the worse the outcome.

Monoclonal antibodies

The second approach involved the use of a genetically engineered monoclonal antibody infliximab (Remicade) in the Anti-TNFα Therapy Against Chronic Heart Failure (ATTACH) phase II study in 150 subjects with moderate to advanced HF. The primary endpoint of the ATTACH trial was also the clinical composite score. Subjects were randomized to receive three separate intravenous infusions of infliximab (5 mg/kg or 10 mg/kg) at baseline, 2, and 4 weeks. Assessment of the clinical composite was made at 14 and 28 weeks. Analysis of the completed study data showed that there was a 21% dose-related increase in death and HF hospitalizations with infliximab when compared with placebo at 14 weeks, and a 26% increase at 28 weeks [81].

Therefore, a careful examination of these two studies shows that anticytokine strategies targeting TNF-α were not neutral, but the results are indeed consistent with a trend of increased mortality and morbidity. Two possible explanations have been offered to clarify these findings [4]. The first is that infliximab and etanercept have intrinsic cytotoxicity. Infliximab exerts its effects, at least in part, by fixing complement in cells that express TNF. Because myocytes express TNF on sarcolemma, complement fixation in the heart could lead to myocyte lysis and further deterioration of cardiac function. Etanercept may also be toxic under certain settings. It has been shown in human studies that etanercept binds to TNF in the peripheral circulation, but this binding is not tight and may dissociate at an extremely fast rate. Rapid dissociation of TNF from etanercept can lead to a paradoxical increase in the duration of TNF bioactivity, opposite of what the therapy was intended to do. The second explanation for worsening HF may be related to the fact that physiologic levels of TNF are cytoprotective and play an important role in tissue remodeling and repair. Excessive antagonism of TNF may, therefore, result in the loss of one or more of its beneficial effects, with consequent loss of homeostasis and resulting in worsening HF. Moreover, the RENAISSANCE MRI remodeling substudy also showed a neutral effect of etanercept on LV structure and function.

Immune modulation therapy

Recently, a novel approach to regulate inflammatory cytokines in the blood has been developed. In this approach, a patient's blood is exposed to controlled oxidative stress in a special device (Celacade) and subsequently administrated intramuscularly. Preliminary experimental studies have demonstrated that this approach may downregulate proinflammatory cytokines and activate several anti-inflammatory cytokines. The hypothesis was tested in the ACCLAIM (Advanced Chronic heart failure Clinical Assessment of Immune Modulation therapy) study [82], a multicenter, randomized, double-blind, placebo-controlled clinical trial in 2,408 NYHA class II to IV HF subjects with LV ejection fraction of 30% or less. The primary endpoint of the study was the combined endpoint of total mortality or cardiovascular hospitalization. Subjects in the ACCLAIM trial were well treated with diuretics (94%), ACE-I (94%), beta blockers (87%), automatic implantable cardioverter defibrillators (26%), and cardiac resynchronization therapy (10.5%). Although the primary endpoint was not different in the placebo and immune modulation therapy groups ($P = .22$), a prespecified subgroup analysis in 689 NYHA class II patients showed that Celacade immunotherapy reduced the risk of mortality or cardiovascular hospitalizations by 39% ($P = .0003$) [83], suggesting that this therapy might be effective in patients who have not reached more advanced stages of HF. The quality of life in the entire study population was significantly improved in the Celacade group ($P = .04$). The procedure was well tolerated, with no significant between-group differences for any serious adverse events. A confirmatory study in NYHA class II patients is being planned.

Vasopressin antagonism

Arginine vasopressin (AVP) activity is increased or inappropriately elevated in patients with HF and contributes to fluid retention and hyponatremia [84,85]. Whereas vasopressin V_{1A} receptors primarily mediate vasoconstriction, direct positive inotropic and mitogenic effects, the V_2 receptors inhibit free water clearance (aquaresis). Agents that antagonize V_{1A} receptors would be expected to reduce vascular tone and the direct mitogenic myocardial effects of AVP. Because V_2 antagonists increase aquaresis, the addition of an AVP V_2 antagonist to standard therapy in patients with congestive HF could represent a novel mechanism to improve free water clearance, thus decreasing the need for diuretic therapy, improving diuretic resistance, reducing the frequency of hyponatremia, and attenuating disease progression. Four agents, three oral selective V_2 antagonists (tolvaptan, lixivaptan, and satavaptan), and one intravenous dual AVP V_{1A}/V_2 antagonist (conivaptan) are under investigation in both HF and hyponatremia. The field has advanced more in hyponatremia, where conivaptan has already received United States Food and Drug Administration approval for intravenouos administration in hospitalized patients with euvolemic or hypervolemic hyponatremia [86].

Tolvaptan has the largest database in HF. Phase II trials have shown that use of tolvaptan is associated with an early and sustained reduction in body weight over 7 to 30 days, consistent with inhibition of an active V_2 receptor-mediated effect on fluid retention. Patients lost weight during the first few days of therapy, but no further weight change was seen thereafter, despite the drug being continued. Tolvaptan administration also tended to normalize serum sodium concentrations in patients with baseline hyponatremia and was not associated with hypokalemia [87,88].

Based on these results, the EVEREST (Efficacy of Vasopressin Antagonism in Heart Failure Outcome Study With Tolvaptan) study was designed to examine whether short-term and long-term blockade of the V_2 receptor with tolvaptan is beneficial in patients with HF and signs and symptoms of volume overload. The results confirmed that tolvaptan, when added to standard therapy including diuretics, improves many—though not all—of the signs and symptoms of HF, as assessed by both subjects and physicians. The reductions in body weight in response to tolvaptan on day 1 were accompanied by significant improvements in subject and physician-assessed dyspnea, orthopnea, fatigue, jugular venous distention, rales, and edema, showed improvements on day 1 and remained better than placebo during the first 3 days or longer. However, despite the improvement in signs and symptoms of HF, no benefit in global clinical status was seen at day 7 or discharge. These effects were achieved without adversely affecting heart rate, blood pressure, or serum electrolytes, and there was no excess of renal failure. Over the long-term, however, tolvaptan treatment had no effect, either favorable or unfavorable, on all-cause mortality or the combined endpoint of cardiovascular mortality or subsequent hospitalization for worsening HF [15]. The drug also had no significant effect on long-term LV remodeling in patients with mild to moderate HF with LV ejection fraction less than 30% [89].

Because selective blockade of the AVP V_2 receptor may cause unopposed activation of the V_{1A} receptor, leading to the deleterious consequences of systemic and coronary vasoconstriction, a dual V_{1A}/V_2 antagonist might be more effective in HF. Although small phase II trials have shown improvement in hemodynamics and urine output after a single intravenous dose of conivaptan [90], no long-term outcome data are available. Thus, although AVP antagonists might be useful in acute HF with or without diuretics, it is unlikely they will have an important role in the management of HF.

Calcium sensitizers

Calcium sensitizers are a new class of inotropic drugs. They improve myocardial performance by directly acting on contractile proteins without increasing intracellular calcium load. Thus, they avoid the undesirable effects of arrhythmias and increase in myocardial oxygen consumption associated with increased intracellular calcium that occurs with other inotropic agents, such as catecholamines and phosphodiesterase-III (PDE) inhibitors.

Two calcium sensitizers have been investigated in patients with HF. Pimobendan, a calcium sensitizer that also exerts a significant inhibition of PDE at clinically relevant doses, significantly increased exercise duration, peak oxygen consumption per unit time (VO_2), and quality of life in 149 patients with moderate to severe HF, over a 12-week period [91]. Its further development has, however, been stopped because of possible deleterious effects on mortality. Levosimendan is a calcium sensitizer with no major inhibition of PDE at clinically relevant doses. It also opens adenosine triphosphate-dependent potassium channels and has vasodilating and cardioprotective effects. In HF patients, levosimendan causes a dose-dependent increase in cardiac output and a decrease in pulmonary capillary wedge pressure. Because levosimendan has an active metabolite, OR-1896, with a half-life of about 80 hours, the duration of the hemodynamic effect significantly exceeds the 1-hour half-life of the parent compound. Three moderate-sized phase II clinical trials (LIDO, RUSSLAN, and CASINO) tested the effects of levosimendan in patients with acute decompensated HF.

Both the RUSSLAN [92] and LIDO [93] trials showed that levosimendan was safe and reduced mortality when compared with placebo and dobutamine, respectively. The results of the CASINO trial [94] have been presented at the American College of Cardiology meeting in 2004 but not published. In this trial, levosimendan also improved survival, compared with dobutamine or placebo, in subjects with acute decompensated HF. These studies were performed in subjects with high filling pressures. In contrast, the two large mortality and morbidity studies (SURVIVE and REVIVE-II) in patients who were hospitalized because of worsening HF did not require filling pressures to be measured.

The SURVIVE (Survival of Patients With Acute Heart Failure in Need of Intravenous Inotropic Support) trial was a randomized, double-blind trial comparing the efficacy and safety of intravenous levosimendan ($n = 664$) or dobutamine ($n = 663$) in subjects hospitalized with acute decompensated HF who required inotropic support [95]. The primary outcome of all-cause mortality at 180 days was no different, with 26% deaths in the levosimendan group and 28% deaths in the dobutamine group ($P = .40$). The other secondary endpoints (all-cause mortality at 31 days, number of days alive and out of the hospital, patient global assessment, patient assessment of dyspnea at 24 hours, and cardiovascular mortality at 180 days) were also not different. There was a higher incidence of cardiac failure in the dobutamine group, but a higher incidence of atrial fibrillation, hypokalemia, and headache in the levosimendan group. Because levosimendan was compared with dobutamine, which is known to increase mortality, a neutral trial raises concerns about the safety of levosimendan.

The REVIVE-II trial was presented at the American Heart Association scientific sessions in 2005 and reported a superior effect of levosimendan on the composite primary outcome,

compared with placebo [96]. However, the details have yet to be published. Thus, until the results of REVIVE-II can be fully scrutinized and placed in the context of all available evidence, we will have to conclude that levosimendan does not have a place in either acute or chronic HF.

Novel agents and approaches under investigation

A number of other and novel agents are being actively investigated, but only a few have reached the stage of testing in phase III clinical trials.

Hydroxymethylglutaryl coenzyme-A reductase inhibitors in heart failure

Hydroxymethylglutaryl coenzyme-A (HMG-CoA) reductase inhibitors (statins) are widely used to modify the lipid profile for primary and secondary prevention of cardiovascular disease. Increasing attention has recently focused on other potentially favorable "pleiotropic" effects that may apply in the setting of HF [97]. Statins have been shown to induce angiogenesis by recruiting bone marrow stem cells [98], reducing levels of inflammatory factors, and improving endothelial function [99,100]. On the other hand, epidemiologic studies have observed a higher risk of adverse events with low levels of low-density lipoprotein cholesterol in patients with HF [101,102]. Statins may diminish the ability of lipoproteins to bind endotoxins, leading to stimulation of proinflammatory cytokines [103], and reduced levels of coenzyme Q10 [104] and selenoproteins [105], which could adversely affect cardiac muscle and function. They also have deleterious interactions with medications commonly used for HF, such as digoxin [106].

Go and colleagues [107] evaluated the association between initiation of statin therapy and risks for death and hospitalization among 24,598 adults diagnosed with HF who had no prior statin use, and found that incident statin use was independently associated with lower risks of death and hospitalization among patients with or without coronary heart disease [107]. Several post-hoc subgroup analyses of clinical trials have found that use of statin therapy was associated with improved survival in patients with ischemic and nonischemic HF [108,109]. However, a recently published CORONA trial (Controlled Rosuvastatin Multinational Study in Heart Failure) found no effect of rosuvastatin on the primary composite outcome of death from cardiovascular causes, nonfatal myocardial infarction, or nonfatal stroke in 5,011 older subjects with systolic heart failure [110]. The GISSI-HF trial (Gruppo Italiano per lo Studio della Sopravvivenza nell'Infarto Micardico – Heart Failure) is currently investigating the effects of rosuvastatin and n-3 polyunsaturated fatty acids on mortality and morbidity in 7,000 subjects with NYHA class II to IV HF of any etiology [111]. The results are expected in 2008 or 2009.

Anemia and heart failure

Anemia is common in patients with HF and is an independent risk factor for worse outcomes [101,112–114]. Although the pathogenesis of anemia in patients with HF is unclear, several mechanisms have been implicated. Impaired renal perfusion with decreased erythropoiesis is probably an important factor. However, there is evidence that erythropoietin levels are increased in HF [115,116], suggesting a relative erythropoietin resistance in this condition. Inflammation has also been implicated: TNF-α and several other proinflammatory cytokines [117], and circulating neutrophils and C-reactive protein, are elevated in HF patients [118]. TNF-α may cause anemia by a number of mechanisms, including inhibition of erythropoietin production in the kidney, preventing erythropoietin from stimulating bone marrow production of erythrocytes and preventing the release of iron from body stores [119]. ACE-inhibitors [120] and angiotensin receptor blockers [114] used in the treatment of HF cause a modest reduction in hemoglobin, probably by inhibiting erythropoietin synthesis, and may contribute to the development of anemia [121]. Although hematinic abnormalities are generally not seen in HF [122], iron deficiency may be common [123] because of impaired metabolism in HF-associated cachexia [124] and aspirin-induced gastrointestinal bleeding. Finally, hemodilution, because of the increase in plasma volume, has been found to be the cause of anemia in nearly half the patients with severe end-stage HF [125]. Thus, multiple mechanisms could cause anemia in patients with HF.

Should we treat anemia in patients with HF? Several small uncontrolled studies have shown that treatment of anemia with erythropoietin was associated with improvements in LV ejection fraction, peak oxygen consumption, NYHA functional class, and a decrease in diuretic requirement [126–128]. However, blood transfusions to increase hemoglobin are associated with an increase

in systemic vascular resistance and blood pressure, and a decrease in cardiac output [129,130]. In patients with chronic kidney disease (CKD) undergoing hemodialysis, raising hematocrit with erythropoietin was associated with an increase in adverse cardiovascular events [131]. More recently, the CHOIR (Corrections of Hemoglobin and Outcomes in Renal Insufficiency) trial showed that treating CKD patients not on hemodialysis, with epoetin alfa targeted to achieve a hemoglobin level of 13.5 g/dL versus 11.3 g/dL, was associated with increased risk of the composite of death, myocardial infarction, hospitalization for congestive HF, and stroke (hazard ratio, 1.34; 95% confidence interval, 1.03 to 1.74; $P = .03$) [132]. These findings therefore raise important concerns about the optimal level of hemoglobin and whether hemoglobin should be raised in patients with HF.

Recently, the results of STAMINA-HeFT (Study of Anemia in Heart Failure–Heart Failure Trial), the largest multicenter, randomized, double-blind, placebo-controlled trial to date evaluating the effect of treating anemia in HF was reported [133]. In this study, 319 subjects with symptomatic HF, LV ejection fraction less than or equal to 40%, and hemoglobin greater than or equal to 9.0 g/dL and less than or equal to 12.5 g/dL, were randomized to placebo or darbepoetin alfa subcutaneously every 2 weeks for 1 year, to achieve a target hemoglobin of 14.0 g/dL plus or minus 1.0 g/dL. The primary endpoint was change from baseline to week 27 in treadmill exercise duration. Secondary endpoints were change from baseline in NYHA class and quality of life at week 27. All cause mortality or first HF hospitalization and all-cause mortality at 1 year was a prespecified efficacy and safety endpoint. At baseline, the median and interquartile range (IQR) hemoglobin was 11.4 (10.9, 12.0) g/dL. At week 27, darbepoetin alfa treatment increased median (IQR) hemoglobin by 1.80 (1.1, 2.5) g/dL (placebo: 0.3 (−0.2, 1.0) g/dL; $P < .001$). Darbepoetin alfa treatment did not significantly improve exercise duration, NYHA class, or quality of life score compared with placebo. A nonsignificant trend was observed toward a lower risk of all-cause mortality or first HF hospitalization at 1 year in darbepoetin alfa-treated subjects, compared with placebo (hazard ratio 0.68; 95% confidence interval 0.43, 1.08; $P = .10$). Adverse events were similar in both treatment groups. The trend of a lower risk of morbidity and mortality, and the safety results of this study have encouraged the conduct of an adequately powered outcome trial RED-HF (Reduction of Events with Darbe-poetin in Heart Failure Trial) for the treatment of anemia in HF. The results of the trial may not be known until 2010.

Summary

Inhibiting the deleterious consequences of activated renin-angiotensin-aldosterone and sympathetic systems with ACE-inhibitors, beta-blockers, and aldosterone receptor antagonists have had an enormous impact on reducing HF mortality and morbidity. These agents currently comprise the "standard of care" of HF treatment. However, extending this paradigm to other activated NH and cytokine systems by stacking multiple NH blockers together has not shown any incremental benefit, and may have deleterious consequences. It must be recognized that all new therapies for HF have to be tested on incremental benefit above the effects achieved by the "standard of care" therapies. There is, therefore, no way to assess whether newer therapies are as effective, or indeed even more effective than either ACE-inhibitors, beta-blockers, or aldosterone blockers. Hence, the disappointing results of recent HF trials is no reflection on the soundness of the neurohormonal hypothesis nor on the effectiveness of the drug being tested, but rather on the strategy of stacking newer drugs on top of the standard of care.

Another fact that needs to be emphasized is that treatment with the standard of care medications and use of devices have resulted in very low mortality rates in clinical trials, which may be difficult to improve upon. Testing the newer agents in higher risk patients may have yielded different results. This notwithstanding, there are numerous examples where clear-cut deleterious consequences of excessive NH and cytokine inhibition are seen. These findings underscore the fact that not all of the body's responses in HF are harmful and need to be blocked. Hence, it does appear that we may have reached a therapeutic ceiling for the neurohormonal approach. Thus, further improvement in the management of HF patients may require new paradigms.

References

[1] Anand IS, Florea VG. Alterations in ventricular structure: role of left ventricular remodeling. In: Mann DL, editor. Heart failure: companion to Braunwald's heart disease. Philadelphia: Saunders; 2002. p. 229–45.

[2] Mann D, Kent R, Parsons B, et al. Adrenergic effects on the biology of the adult mammalian cardiocyte. Circulation 1992;85:790–804.

[3] Tan LB, Jalil JE, Pick R, et al. Cardiac myocyte necrosis induced by angiotensin II. Circ Res 1991; 69(5):1185–95.

[4] Mann DL. Inflammatory mediators and the failing heart: past, present, and the foreseeable future. Circ Res 2002;91(11):988–98.

[5] Anand IS, Chandrashekhar Y. Neurohormonal responses in congestive heart failure: effect of ACE inhibitors in randomized controlled clinical trials. In: Dhalla NS, Singhal PK, Beamish RE, editors. Heart hypertrophy and failure. Boston: Kluwer Academic Publishers; 1996. p. 487–501.

[6] Anand IS, Fisher LD, Chiang YT, et al. Changes in brain natriuretic peptide and norepinephrine over time and mortality and morbidity in Val-HeF. Circulation 2003;107:1276–81.

[7] CONSENSUS Trial Study Group. Effects of enalapril on mortality in severe congestive heart failure. Results of the Cooperative North Scandinavian Enalapril Survival Study (CONSENSUS). N Engl J Med 1987;316(23):1429–35.

[8] Effect of enalapril on survival in patients with reduced left ventricular ejection fractions and congestive heart failure. The SOLVD Investigators. N Engl J Med 1991;325(5):293–302.

[9] The MERIT-HF Investigators. Effect of metoprolol CR/XL in chronic heart failure: Metoprolol CR/XL Randomised Intervention Trial in Congestive Heart Failure (MERIT-HF). Lancet 1999;353:2001–7.

[10] Packer M, Coats AJ, Fowler MB, et al. Effect of carvedilol on survival in severe chronic heart failure. N Engl J Med 2001;344(22):1651–8.

[11] Pitt B, Zannad F, Remme WJ, et al. The effect of spironolactone on morbidity and mortality in patients with severe heart failure. Randomized Aldactone evaluation study investigators. N Engl J Med 1999;341(10):709–17.

[12] Cohn JN, Tognoni G. A randomized trial of the angiotensin-receptor blocker valsartan in chronic heart failure. N Engl J Med 2001;345(23):1667–75.

[13] Packer M, McMurray J, Massie BM, et al. Clinical effects of endothelin receptor antagonism with bosentan in patients with severe chronic heart failure: results of a pilot study. J Card Fail 2005; 11(1):12–20.

[14] Packer M, Califf RM, Konstam MA, et al. Comparison of omapatrilat and enalapril in patients with chronic heart failure: the Omapatrilat Versus Enalapril Randomized Trial of Utility in Reducing Events (OVERTURE). Circulation 2002;106(8): 920–6.

[15] Konstam MA, Gheorghiade M, Burnett JC Jr, et al. Effects of oral tolvaptan in patients

hospitalized for worsening heart failure: the EVEREST Outcome Trial. JAMA 2007;297(12): 1319–31.

[16] Anand IS, McMurray JJ, Cohn JN, et al. Long-term Effects of Darusentan on LV Remodeling and Clinical Outcomes—The EndothelinA Receptor Antagonist Trial in Heart Failure (EARTH). Lancet 2004;364(9431):347–54.

[17] The CIBIS II Investigators. The Cardiac Insufficiency Bisoprolol Study II (CIBIS-II): a randomised trial. Lancet 1999;353(9146):9–13.

[18] Hall SA, Cigarroa CG, Marcoux L, et al. Time course of improvement in left ventricular function, mass and geometry in patients with congestive heart failure treated with beta-adrenergic blockade. J Am Coll Cardiol 1995;25(5):1154–61.

[19] Doherty NI, Seelos K, Suzuki J-I, et al. Application of cine nuclear magnetic resonance imaging for sequential evaluation of response to angiotensin-converting enzyme inhibitor therapy in dilated cardiomyopathy. J Am Coll Cardiol 1992;19: 1294–302.

[20] Cohn JN, Levine TB, Olivari MT, et al. Plasma norepinephrine as a guide to prognosis in patients with chronic congestive heart failure. N Engl J Med 1984;311(13):819–23.

[21] Bristow MR, Gilbert EM, Abraham WT, et al. Carvedilol produces dose-related improvements in left ventricular function and survival in subjects with chronic heart failure. MOCHA Investigators. Circulation 1996;94(11):2807–16.

[22] Swedberg K, Bristow MR, Cohn JN, et al. Effects of sustained-release moxonidine, an imidazoline agonist, on plasma norepinephrine in patients with chronic heart failure. Circulation 2002;105(15): 1797–803.

[23] Cohn JN, Pfeffer MA, Rouleau J, et al. Adverse mortality effect of central sympathetic inhibition with sustained-release moxonidine in patients with heart failure (MOXCON). Eur J Heart Fail 2003;5(5):659–67.

[24] The BEST Investigators. A trial of the beta-blocker bucindolol in patients with advanced chronic heart failure. N Engl J Med 2001; 344(22):1659–67.

[25] Bristow M, Krause-Steinrauf H, Abraham WT, et al. Sympatholytic effect of bucindolol adversely affected survival, and was disproportionately observed in the class IV subgroup of BEST. Circulation 2001;104(17):II-755.

[26] The SOLVD Investigators. Effect of enalapril on mortality and the development of heart failure in asymptomatic patients with reduced left ventricular ejection fractions. N Engl J Med 1992;327(10): 685–91.

[27] Pfeffer MA, Braunwald E, Moye LA, et al. Effect of captopril on mortality and morbidity in patients with left ventricular dysfunction after myocardial infarction. Results of the survival and ventricular

enlargement trial. N Engl J Med 1992;327(10): 669–77.

[28] The AIRE Study Investigators. Effect of ramipril on mortality and morbidity of survivors of acute myocardial infarction with clinical evidence of heart failure. Lancet 1993;342(8875):821–8.

[29] Kober L, Torp-Pedersen C, Carlsen JE, et al. A clinical trial of the angiotensin-converting-enzyme inhibitor trandolapril in patients with left ventricular dysfunction after myocardial infarction. Trandolapril Cardiac Evaluation (TRACE) Study Group. N Engl J Med 1995;333(25):1670–6.

[30] St. John Sutton M, Pfeffer MA, Plappert T, et al. Quantitative two-dimensional echocardiographic measurements are major predictors of adverse cardiovascular events after acute myocardial infarction. The protective effects of captopril. Circulation 1994;89(1):68–75.

[31] Greenberg B, Quinones MA, Koilpillai C, et al. Effects of long-term enalapril therapy on cardiac structure and function in patients with left ventricular dysfunction. Results of the SOLVD echocardiography substudy. Circulation 1995;91(10):2573–81.

[32] Packer M, Poole-Wilson PA, Armstrong PW, et al. Comparative effects of low and high doses of the angiotensin-converting enzyme inhibitor, lisinopril, on morbidity and mortality in chronic heart failure. ATLAS Study Group. Circulation 1999; 100(23):2312–8.

[33] Nanas JN, Alexopoulos G, Anastasiou-Nana MI, et al. Outcome of patients with congestive heart failure treated with standard versus high doses of enalapril: a multicenter study. High Enalapril Dose Study Group. J Am Coll Cardiol 2000; 36(7):2090–5.

[34] Tang WH, Vagelos RH, Yee YG, et al. Neurohormonal and clinical responses to high- versus low-dose enalapril therapy in chronic heart failure. J Am Coll Cardiol 2002;39(1):70–8.

[35] Kawamura M, Imanashi M, Matsushima Y, et al. Circulating angiotensin II levels under repeated administration of lisinopril in normal subjects. Clin Exp Pharmacol Physiol 1992;19(8):547–53.

[36] Jorde UP, Ennezat PV, Lisker J, et al. Maximally recommended doses of angiotensin-converting enzyme (ACE) inhibitors do not completely prevent ACE-mediated formation of angiotensin II in chronic heart failure. Circulation 2000;101(8): 844–6.

[37] Pfeffer MA, Swedberg K, Granger CB, et al. Effects of candesartan on mortality and morbidity in patients with chronic heart failure: the CHARM-Overall programme. Lancet 2003;362(9386): 759–66.

[38] Yusuf S, Pfeffer MA, Swedberg K, et al. Effects of candesartan in patients with chronic heart failure and preserved left-ventricular ejection fraction: the CHARM-Preserved Trial. Lancet 2003; 362(9386):777–81.

[39] Granger CB, McMurray JJ, Yusuf S, et al. Effects of candesartan in patients with chronic heart failure and reduced left-ventricular systolic function intolerant to angiotensin-converting-enzyme inhibitors: the CHARM-Alternative trial. Lancet 2003; 362(9386):772–6.

[40] McMurray JJ, Ostergren J, Swedberg K, et al. Effects of candesartan in patients with chronic heart failure and reduced left-ventricular systolic function taking angiotensin-converting-enzyme inhibitors: the CHARM-Added trial. Lancet 2003; 362(9386):767–71.

[41] Pfeffer MA, McMurray JJ, Velazquez EJ, et al. Valsartan, captopril, or both in myocardial infarction complicated by heart failure, left ventricular dysfunction, or both. N Engl J Med 2003;349(20): 1893–906.

[42] Maggioni AP, Anand I, Gottlieb SO, et al. Effects of valsartan on morbidity and mortality in patients with heart failure not receiving angiotensin-converting enzyme inhibitors. J Am Coll Cardiol 2002;40(8):1414–21.

[43] Wong M, Staszewsky L, Latini R, et al. Valsartan benefits left ventricular structure and function in heart failure: Val-HeFT echocardiographic study. J Am Coll Cardiol 2002;40(5):970–5.

[44] Weber K, Brilla C, Janicki J. Myocardial fibrosis: functional significance and regulatory factors. Cardiovasc Res 1993;27:341–8.

[45] Brilla CG, Matsubara LS, Weber KT. Anti-aldosterone treatment and the prevention of myocardial fibrosis in primary and secondary hyperaldosteronism. J Mol Cell Cardiol 1993;25(5):563–75.

[46] Young M, Fullerton M, Dilley R, et al. Mineralocorticoids, hypertension, and cardiac fibrosis. J Clin Invest 1994;93(6):2578–83.

[47] Sanders LL, Melby JC. Aldosterone and the edema of congestive heart failure. Arch Intern Med 1964; 113:331–41.

[48] Pitt B, Remme W, Zannad F, et al. Eplerenone, a selective aldosterone blocker, in patients with left ventricular dysfunction after myocardial infarction. N Engl J Med 2003;348(14):1309–21.

[49] Hayashi M, Tsutamoto T, Wada A, et al. Immediate administration of mineralocorticoid receptor antagonist spironolactone prevents post-infarct left ventricular remodeling associated with suppression of a marker of myocardial collagen synthesis in patients with first anterior acute myocardial infarction. Circulation 2003;107(20): 2559–65.

[50] Cai H, Harrison DG. Endothelial dysfunction in cardiovascular diseases: the role of oxidant stress. Circ Res 2000;87(10):840–4.

[51] Drexler H. Nitric oxide synthases in the failing human heart: a doubled-edged sword? Circulation 1999;99(23):2972–5.

[52] Liu YH, Xu J, Yang XP, et al. Effect of ACE inhibitors and angiotensin II type 1 receptor antagonists on endothelial NO synthase knockout mice with heart failure. Hypertension 2002;39(2 Pt 2):375–81.

[53] Jones SP, Greer JJ, van Haperen R, et al. Endothelial nitric oxide synthase overexpression attenuates congestive heart failure in mice. Proc Natl Acad Sci U S A 2003;100(8):4891–6.

[54] Scherrer-Crosbie M, Ullrich R, Bloch KD, et al. Endothelial nitric oxide synthase limits left ventricular remodeling after myocardial infarction in mice. Circulation 2001;104(11):1286–91.

[55] Dixon LJ, Morgan DR, Hughes SM, et al. Functional consequences of endothelial nitric oxide synthase uncoupling in congestive cardiac failure. Circulation 2003;107(13):1725–8.

[56] Drexler H, Hayoz D, Munzel T, et al. Endothelial function in chronic congestive heart failure. Am J Cardiol 1992;69(19):1596–601.

[57] Kubo SH, Rector TS, Bank AJ, et al. Endothelium-dependent vasodilation is attenuated in patients with heart failure. Circulation 1991;84(4):1589–96.

[58] Munzel T, Harrison DG. Increased superoxide in heart failure: a biochemical baroreflex gone awry. Circulation 1999;100(3):216–8.

[59] Mohri M, Egashira K, Tagawa T, et al. Basal release of nitric oxide is decreased in the coronary circulation in patients with heart failure. Hypertension 1997;30(1 Pt 1):50–6.

[60] Hare JM, Givertz MM, Creager MA, et al. Increased sensitivity to nitric oxide synthase inhibition in patients with heart failure: potentiation of beta-adrenergic inotropic responsiveness. Circulation 1998;97(2):161–6.

[61] Cohn JN, Archibald DG, Ziesche S, et al. Effect of vasodilator therapy on mortality in chronic congestive heart failure. Results of a Veterans Administration Cooperative Study. N Engl J Med 1986; 314(24):1547–52.

[62] Taylor AL, Ziesche S, Yancy C, et al. Combination of isosorbide dinitrate and hydralazine in blacks with heart failure. N Engl J Med 2004;351(20): 2049–57.

[63] Cohn JN, Tam SW, Anand IS, et al. Isosorbide dinitrate and hydralazine in a fixed-dose combination produces further regression of left ventricular remodeling in a well-treated black population with heart failure: results from A-HeFT. J Card Fail 2007;13(5):331–9.

[64] Cintron G, Johnson G, Francis G, et al. Prognostic significance of serial changes in left ventricular ejection fraction in patients with congestive heart failure. Circulation 1993; 87(Suppl 6):VI17–23.

[65] Yanagisawa M, Kurihara H, Kimura S, et al. A novel potent vasoconstrictor peptide produced by vascular endothelial cells. Nature 1988; 332(6163):411–5.

[66] Haynes WG, Webb DJ. Contribution of endogenous generation of endothelin-1 to basal vascular tone. Lancet 1994;344(8926):852–4.

[67] Stewart DJ, Cernacek P, Costello KB, et al. Elevated endothelin-1 in heart failure and loss of normal response to postural change. Circulation 1992;85(2):510–7.

[68] McMurray JJ, Ray SG, Abdullah I, et al. Plasma endothelin in chronic heart failure. Circulation 1992;85(4):1374–9.

[69] Omland T, Lie RT, Aakvaag A, et al. Plasma endothelin determination as a prognostic indicator of 1-year mortality after acute myocardial infarction. Circulation 1994;89(4):1573–9.

[70] Fukuchi M, Giaid A. Expression of endothelin-1 and endothelin-converting enzyme-1 mRNAs and proteins in failing human hearts. J Cardiovasc Pharmacol 1998;31(Suppl 1):S421–3.

[71] Sakai S, Miyauchi T, Kobayashi M, et al. Inhibition of myocardial endothelin pathway improves long-term survival in heart failure. Nature 1996; 384(6607):353–5.

[72] Sutsch G, Kiowski W, Yan XW, et al. Short-term oral endothelin-receptor antagonist therapy in conventionally treated patients with symptomatic severe chronic heart failure. Circulation 1998; 98(21):2262–8.

[73] Luscher TF, Enseleit F, Pacher R, et al. Hemodynamic and neurohumoral effects of selective endothelin A (ET(A)) receptor blockade in chronic heart failure: the Heart Failure ET(A) Receptor Blockade Trial (HEAT). Circulation 2002; 106(21):2666–72.

[74] Wada A, Tsutamoto T, Fukai D, et al. Comparison of the effects of selective endothelin ETA and ETB receptor antagonists in congestive heart failure. J Am Coll Cardiol 1997;30(5):1385–92.

[75] Mann DL. Mechanisms and models in heart failure: a combinatorial approach. Circulation 1999;100(9): 999–1008.

[76] Kapadia S, Torre-Amione G, Yokoyama T, et al. Soluble TNF binding proteins modulate the negative inotropic properties of TNF-alpha in vitro. Am J Physiol 1995;268(2 Pt 2):H517–25.

[77] Deswal A, Bozkurt B, Seta Y, et al. Safety and efficacy of a soluble P75 tumor necrosis factor receptor (Enbrel, etanercept) in patients with advanced heart failure. Circulation 1999;99(25):3224–6.

[78] Bozkurt B, Torre-Amione G, Warren MS, et al. Results of targeted anti-tumor necrosis factor therapy with etanercept (ENBREL) in patients with advanced heart failure. Circulation 2001;103(8): 1044–7.

[79] Wood S. RENEWAL trial: no improvement in CHF with etanercept. HeartWire News 2002. Available at: http://www.theheart.org. Accessed August 15, 2002.

[80] Mann DL, McMurray JJ, Packer M, et al. Targeted anticytokine therapy in patients with chronic heart failure: results of the Randomized Etanercept Worldwide Evaluation (RENEWAL). Circulation 2004;109(13):1594–602.

[81] Packer M, Chung E, Batra S, et al. Randomized placebo-controlled dose-ranging trial of infliximab, a monoclonal antibody to tumor necrosis factor-alpha, in moderate to severe heart failure. Presented at the Annual Meeting of HFSA. Boca Raton, FL, September 25, 2002.

[82] Torre-Amione G, Bourge RC, Colucci WS, et al. A study to assess the effects of a broad-spectrum immune modulatory therapy on mortality and morbidity in patients with chronic heart failure: the ACCLAIM trial rationale and design. Can J Cardiol 2007;23(5):369–76.

[83] Torre-Amione G. Advanced Chronic Heart Failure Clinical Assessment of Immune Modulation Therapy (ACCLAIM) trial: a placebo-controlled randomised trial. Lancet 2008;371(9608):228–36.

[84] Anand I, Ferrari R, Kalra G, et al. Edema of cardiac origin. Studies of body water and sodium, renal function, hemodynamic indexes, and plasma hormones in untreated congestive cardiac failure. Circulation 1989;80:299–305.

[85] Goldsmith SR, Gheorghiade M. Vasopressin antagonism in heart failure. J Am Coll Cardiol 2005;46(10):1785–91.

[86] Ghali JK, Koren MJ, Taylor JR, et al. Efficacy and safety of oral conivaptan: a V1A/V2 vasopressin receptor antagonist, assessed in a randomized, placebo-controlled trial in patients with euvolemic or hypervolemic hyponatremia. J Clin Endocrinol Metab 2006;91(6):2145–52.

[87] Gheorghiade M, Gattis WA, O'Connor CM, et al. Effects of tolvaptan, a vasopressin antagonist, in patients hospitalized with worsening heart failure: a randomized controlled trial. JAMA 2004; 291(16):1963–71.

[88] Gheorghiade M, Niazi I, Ouyang J, et al. Vasopressin V2-receptor blockade with tolvaptan in patients with chronic heart failure: results from a double-blind, randomized trial. Circulation 2003;107(21): 2690–6.

[89] Udelson JE, McGrew FA, Flores E, et al. Multicenter, randomized, double-blind, placebo-controlled study on the effect of oral tolvaptan on left ventricular dilation and function in patients with heart failure and systolic dysfunction. J Am Coll Cardiol 2007;49(22):2151–9.

[90] Udelson JE, Smith WB, Hendrix GH, et al. Acute hemodynamic effects of conivaptan, a dual V(1A) and V(2) vasopressin receptor antagonist, in patients with advanced heart failure. Circulation 2001;104(20):2417–23.

[91] Kubo SH, Gollub S, Bourge R, et al. Beneficial effects of pimobendan on exercise tolerance and quality of life in patients with heart failure. Results of a multicenter trial. The Pimobendan Multicenter Research Group. Circulation 1992;85(3):942–9.

[92] Moiseyev VS, Poder P, Andrejevs N, et al. Safety and efficacy of a novel calcium sensitizer, levosimendan, in patients with left ventricular failure

due to an acute myocardial infarction. A randomized, placebo-controlled, double-blind study (RUSSLAN). Eur Heart J 2002;23(18):1422–32.

[93] Follath F, Cleland JG, Just H, et al. Efficacy and safety of intravenous levosimendan compared with dobutamine in severe low-output heart failure (the LIDO study): a randomised double-blind trial. Lancet 2002;360(9328):196–202.

[94] Cleland JG, Ghosh J, Freemantle N, et al. Clinical trials update and cumulative meta-analyses from the American College of Cardiology: WATCH, SCD-HeFT, DINAMIT, CASINO, INSPIRE, STRATUS-US, RIO-Lipids and cardiac resynchronisation therapy in heart failure. Eur J Heart Fail 2004;6(4):501–8.

[95] Mebazaa A, Nieminen MS, Packer M, et al. Levosimendan vs dobutamine for patients with acute decompensated heart failure: the SURVIVE Randomized Trial. JAMA 2007;297(17):1883–91.

[96] Cleland JG, Freemantle N, Coletta AP, et al. Clinical trials update from the American Heart Association: REPAIR-AMI, ASTAMI, JELIS, MEGA, REVIVE-II, SURVIVE, and PROACTIVE. Eur J Heart Fail 2006;8(1):105–10.

[97] Bohm M, Hjalmarson A, Kjekshus J, et al. Heart failure and statins—why do we need a clinical trial? Z Kardiol 2005;94(4):223–30.

[98] Urbich C, Dimmeler S. Risk factors for coronary artery disease, circulating endothelial progenitor cells, and the role of HMG-CoA reductase inhibitors. Kidney Int 2005;67(5):1672–6.

[99] Strey CH, Young JM, Molyneux SL, et al. Endothelium-ameliorating effects of statin therapy and coenzyme Q10 reductions in chronic heart failure. Atherosclerosis 2005;179(1):201–6.

[100] Tousoulis D, Antoniades C, Bosinakou E, et al. Effects of atorvastatin on reactive hyperemia and inflammatory process in patients with congestive heart failure. Atherosclerosis 2005;178(2):359–63.

[101] Horwich TB, Fonarow GC, Hamilton MA, et al. Anemia is associated with worse symptoms, greater impairment in functional capacity and a significant increase in mortality in patients with advanced heart failure. J Am Coll Cardiol 2002;39(11): 1780–6.

[102] Rauchhaus M, Clark AL, Doehner W, et al. The relationship between cholesterol and survival in patients with chronic heart failure. J Am Coll Cardiol 2003;42(11):1933–40.

[103] Rauchhaus M, Coats AJ, Anker SD. The endotoxin-lipoprotein hypothesis. Lancet 2000;356(9233): 930–3.

[104] Rundek T, Naini A, Sacco R, et al. Atorvastatin decreases the coenzyme Q10 level in the blood of patients at risk for cardiovascular disease and stroke. Arch Neurol 2004;61(6):889–92.

[105] Moosmann B, Behl C. Selenoprotein synthesis and side-effects of statins. Lancet 2004;363(9412): 892–4.

[106] Bellosta S, Paoletti R, Corsini A. Safety of statins: focus on clinical pharmacokinetics and drug interactions. Circulation 2004;109(23 Suppl 1):III50–7.

[107] Go AS, Lee WY, Yang J, et al. Statin therapy and risks for death and hospitalization in chronic heart failure. JAMA 2006;296(17):2105–11.

[108] Horwich TB, MacLellan WR, Fonarow GC. Statin therapy is associated with improved survival in ischemic and non-ischemic heart failure. J Am Coll Cardiol 2004;43(4):642–8.

[109] Krum H, Latini R, Maggioni AP, et al. Statins and symptomatic chronic systolic heart failure: a post-hoc analysis of 5010 patients enrolled in Val-HeFT. Int J Cardiol 2007;119(1):48–53.

[110] Kjekshus J, Apetrei E, Barrios V, et al. Rosuvastatin in older patients with systolic heart failure. N Engl J Med 2007;357(22):2248–61.

[111] Tavazzi L, Tognoni G, Franzosi MG, et al. Rationale and design of the GISSI heart failure trial: a large trial to assess the effects of n-3 polyunsaturated fatty acids and rosuvastatin in symptomatic congestive heart failure. Eur J Heart Fail 2004; 6(5):635–41.

[112] Cromie N, Lee C, Struthers AD. Anaemia in chronic heart failure: what is its frequency in the UK and its underlying causes? Heart 2002;87(4): 377–8.

[113] Ezekowitz JA, McAlister FA, Armstrong PW. Anemia is common in heart failure and is associated with poor outcomes: insights from a cohort of 12,065 patients with new-onset heart failure. Circulation 2003;107(2):223–5.

[114] Anand IS, Kuskowski MA, Rector TS, et al. Anemia and change in hemoglobin over time related to mortality and morbidity in patients with chronic heart failure: results from Val-HeFT. Circulation 2005;112(8):1121–7.

[115] George J, Patal S, Wexler D, et al. Circulating erythropoietin levels and prognosis in patients with congestive heart failure: comparison with neurohormonal and inflammatory markers. Arch Intern Med 2005;165(11):1304–9.

[116] Volpe M, Tritto C, Testa U, et al. Blood levels of erythropoietin in congestive heart failure and correlation with clinical, hemodynamic, and hormonal profiles. Am J Cardiol 1994;74(5):468–73.

[117] Deswal A, Petersen NJ, Feldman AM, et al. Cytokines and cytokine receptors in advanced heart failure: an analysis of the cytokine database from the Vesnarinone trial (VEST). Circulation 2001; 103(16):2055–9.

[118] Anand IS, Latini R, Florea VG, et al. C-reactive protein in heart failure: prognostic value and the effect of valsartan. Circulation 2005;112(10): 1428–34.

[119] Goicoechea M, Martin J, de Sequera P, et al. Role of cytokines in the response to erythropoietin in hemodialysis patients. Kidney Int 1998;54(4): 1337–43.

[120] Alaattin Y, Naci C, Vakur A, et al. Comparison of the effects of enalapril and losartan on posttransplantation erythrocytosis in renal transplant reciepients: Prospective randomized study. Transplantation 2001;72(3):542–5.

[121] Albitar S, Genin R, Fen-Chong M, et al. High dose enalapril impairs the response to erythropoietin treatment in haemodialysis patients. Nephrol Dial Transplant 1998;13(5):1206–10.

[122] Witte KK, Desilva R, Chattopadhyay S, et al. Are hematinic deficiencies the cause of anemia in chronic heart failure? Am Heart J 2004;147(5): 924–30.

[123] Nanas JN, Matsouka C, Karageorgopoulos D, et al. Etiology of anemia in patients with advanced heart failure. J Am Coll Cardiol 2006;48(12): 2485–9.

[124] Anker SD, Chua TP, Ponikowski P, et al. Hormonal changes and catabolic/anabolic imbalance in chronic heart failure and their importance for cardiac cachexia. Circulation 1997;96(2): 526–34.

[125] Androne AS, Katz SD, Lund L, et al. Hemodilution is common in patients with advanced heart failure. Circulation 2003;107(2):226–9.

[126] Mancini DM, Katz SD, Lang CC, et al. Effect of erythropoietin on exercise capacity in patients with moderate to severe chronic heart failure. Circulation 2003;107(2):294–9.

[127] Silverberg DS, Wexler D, Blum M, et al. The use of subcutaneous erythropoietin and intravenous iron for the treatment of the anemia of severe, resistant congestive heart failure improves cardiac and renal function and functional cardiac class, and markedly reduces hospitalizations. J Am Coll Cardiol 2000;35(7):1737–44.

[128] Silverberg DS, Wexler D, Sheps D, et al. The effect of correction of mild anemia in severe, resistant congestive heart failure using subcutaneous erythropoietin and intravenous iron: a randomized controlled study. J Am Coll Cardiol 2001;37(7): 1775–80.

[129] Anand IS, Chandrashekhar Y, Ferrari R, et al. Pathogenesis of oedema in chronic severe anaemia: studies of body water and sodium, renal function, haemodynamic variables, and plasma hormones. Br Heart J 1993;70(4):357–62.

[130] Anand IS, Chandrashekhar Y, Wander GS, et al. Endothelium-derived relaxing factor is important in mediating the high output state in chronic severe anemia. J Am Coll Cardiol 1995;25(6):1402–7.

[131] Besarab A, Bolton WK, Browne JK, et al. The effects of normal as compared with low hematocrit values in patients with cardiac disease who are receiving hemodialysis and epoetin. N Engl J Med 1998;339(9):584–90.

[132] Singh AK, Szczech L, Tang KL, et al. Correction of anemia with epoetin alfa in chronic kidney disease. N Engl J Med 2006;355(20):2085–98.

[133] Ghali JK, Anand IS, Abraham WT, et al. Randomized Double-Blind Trial of Darbepoetin alfa in Patients With Symptomatic Heart Failure and Anemia. Circulation. January 14, 2008; [epub ahead of print].

ELSEVIER
SAUNDERS

CARDIOLOGY
CLINICS

Cardiol Clin 26 (2008) 73–77

Angiotensin-Converting Enzyme Inhibitor and/or Angiotensin Receptor Antagonist for the Postmyocardial Infarction Patient

Robert L. Scott, MD, PhD, FACC

Mayo Clinic Specialty Building, Mayo Clinic Arizona, 5779 East Mayo Boulevard, Phoenix, AZ 85054

Coronary artery disease is a major cause of cardiovascular morbidity and mortality in the United States. Much of the pathology that is perpetuated with coronary artery disease is mediated through neurohormonal influences. In fact, most therapeutic agents that have been found to be effective in the treatment of various aspects of cardiovascular disease either attenuate or augment key neurohormonal influences [1].

Nowhere is the relationship of neurohormonal influence more evident than in the patient who has left ventricular dysfunction. For the sake of clarification, in this article left ventricular dysfunction is equated with systolic dysfunction unless otherwise mentioned. The key neurohormonal mediators of cardiovascular pathology include but are not limited to the following:

1. Renin
2. Angiotensin II
3. Norepinephrine
4. Endothelin
5. Aldosterone

The levels of these key neurohormones increase commensurate with worsening left ventricular dysfunction. The earliest clinical trials looking at patients who had severe left ventricular dysfunction treated with drugs that specifically inhibit angiotensin II, arguably the most potent vasoconstrictor in the body, demonstrated a significant reduction in mortality from worsening heart failure [2]. The benefits associated with the use of angiotensin-converting enzyme (ACE-I) are present in patients who have left ventricular dysfunction regardless of the origin of disease.

Box 1 outlines several known causes of left ventricular dysfunction. The cause of disease often varies with the demographics of the population in question. African Americans who have left ventricular dysfunction tend to have a higher prevalence of hypertensive heart disease as the cause of disease, whereas whites tend to have a greater percentage of coronary artery disease as the cause of left ventricular dysfunction. In all the populations compared, the overall morbidity and mortality from left ventricular dysfunction is higher among those who have coronary artery disease.

In patients who have left ventricular dysfunction and known coronary artery disease, the use of ACE-I is associated with an improvement in morbidity as well as a reduction in sudden cardiac death [3]. Sudden cardiac death is a catastrophic complication of left ventricular dysfunction, and patients who have coronary artery disease are at particular risk despite optimal medical management. Although the most robust data demonstrating a reduction from sudden cardiac death are in association with beta-blocker therapy, one cannot discount the importance of ACE-I therapy in patients who have left ventricular dysfunction.

The clinical efficacy of ACE-I therapy in patients who have left ventricular dysfunction is predicated on robust prospective, randomized clinical trial data showing a consistent reduction in mortality. As demonstrated in Table 1, the reduction in mortality in ACE-I use seems to be a class effect, in that efficacy is noted with several different agents.

E-mail address: scott.robert@mayo.edu

> ### Box 1. Causes of left ventricular dysfunction
>
> Coronary artery disease
> Hypertension
> Idiopathic causes
> Viral infections
> Thyroid disorder
> Chemotherapeutic agents
> Cocaine/methamphetamine use

The Survival and Ventricular Enlargement (SAVE) trial was a landmark trial demonstrating the efficacy of ACE-I use among patients who had left ventricular dysfunction after myocardial infarction [4]. A total of 2230 patients who had left ventricular dysfunction (ejection fraction < 40%) 3 to 16 days after myocardial infarction were assigned randomly to receive captopril or placebo. The captopril group demonstrated lower total mortality as well a lower incidence of fatal or nonfatal major cardiovascular events. The reduction in risk was 21% (95% confidence interval [CI], 5%–35%; $P = .014$) for death from cardiovascular causes, 37% (95% CI, 20%–50%; P < 0.001) for the development of severe heart failure, 22% (95% CI, 4%–37%; $P = .019$) for congestive heart failure requiring

Table 1
Clinical trials demonstrating effectiveness of drugs acting on the renin-angiotensin-aldosterone system

Trial	No. of patients	Comparative agent versus placebo	Impact on mortality (%)
CONSENSUS[a] [2]	253	Enalapril	↓ 27
SOLVD[a] [18,19]	2569	Enalapril	↓ 16
RALES[a] [20]	1663	Spironolactone	↓ 30
SAVE[b] [4]	2231	Captopril	↓ 19
AIRE[b] [7]	2006	Ramipril	↓ 27
TRACE[b] [6]	1749	Trandolapril	↓ 22
HOPE[c] [21]	9297	Ramipril	↓ 16

Abbreviations: HOPE, Heart Outcomes Prevention Evaluation trial; RALES, Randomized Aldactone Evaluation Study; SOLVD, Studies of Left Ventricular Dysfunction.
[a] Heart failure.
[b] After myocardial infarction.
[c] Vasculature.

hospitalization, and 25% (95% CI, 5%–40%; $P = .015$) for recurrent myocardial infarction.

Many of the benefits noted in the SAVE trial came from lessons learned in the Cooperative New Scandinavian Enalapril Survival Study II (CONSENSUS II) trial [5]. In the CONSENSUS II trial, patients who had acute myocardial infarction received intravenous enalapril within 1 hour of presentation if their systolic blood pressure was higher than 100 mm Hg. Subsequently enalapril was taken orally and continued for 6 months. Therapy had to be changed because of worsening heart failure in 30% of the placebo group and 27% of the enalapril group (P < 0.006). Early hypotension (systolic pressure < 90 mm Hg or diastolic pressure < 50 mm Hg) occurred in 12% of the enalapril group and in 3% of the placebo group (P < 0.001). Given the potential of an adverse effect with intravenous enalapril administered so early in presentation, ACE-I therapy was initiated between day 3 and 16 in the SAVE trial.

The observed benefits do not seem to be unique to either captopril or enalapril, as evidenced by similar reductions in cardiac events in the Trial of the Angiotensin-Converting Enzyme (TRACE) study of trandolapril and the Acute Infarction Ramipril Efficacy (AIRE) trial [6,7]. In the AIRE trial, a total of 2006 patients who had heart failure at the time of presentation with an acute myocardial infarction were assigned randomly to either placebo or ramipril between days 3 and 10. Patients were excluded if the investigator considered their congestive symptoms severe enough to require starting ACE-I therapy. The observed risk reduction in total mortality was 27% ($P = 0.002$). The benefits of ACE-I therapy in patients who have acute myocardial infarction with left ventricular dysfunction are not limited to those patients who receive either thrombolytics or beta-blocker therapy.

One unique question is whether ACE-I therapy shows long-term benefit in patients who have acute myocardial infarction with preserved left ventricular function. The Survival of Myocardial Infarction Long-term Evaluation (SMILE) - ISCHEMIA study sought to answer that important question [8]. A total of 349 patients who had preserved ejection fraction (> 40%) after myocardial infarction were assigned randomly to the ACE-I zofenopril or placebo. The goal was to investigate the effects of ACE-I on relieving the ischemic burden in patients who had preserved left ventricular function after infarction. Patients were enrolled within 1 to 6 weeks after infarction. The primary end point was assessed by combining the occurrence of significant ST-T abnormalities on ambulatory ECG, ECG abnormalities or symptoms of angina during a standard exercise test, recurrence of myocardial infarction, and need for revascularization procedures for angina. The primary end point occurred in 20.3% of the zofenopril-treated patients and in 35.9% of the placebo-treated patients ($P - .001$).

Similarly, the European Trial on Reduction of Cardiac Events with Perindopril in Patients with Stable Coronary Artery Disease (EUROPA) also evaluated the reduction of cardiac events in patients who had stable coronary arteries [9]. In this trial 12,218 patients who had coronary artery disease documented by prior myocardial infarction or revascularization were assigned randomly to either perindopril or placebo. The cohort had no evidence of either congestive failure or poorly controlled hypertension. The perindopril-treated patients had a significant reduction in cardiovascular death, myocardial infarction, cardiac arrest, acute coronary syndromes, and development of heart failure.

Although it is clear that ACE-I therapy attenuates the effects of angiotensin II, conveying favorable cardiovascular benefits, some individuals are intolerant of this class of medication [10]. The most common form of ACE-I intolerance is the "ACE-I cough," which is thought to be related to excessive bradykinin production. In individuals who are intolerant of ACE-I, angiotensin receptor antagonists (ARB) have emerged as a highly effective class of antihypertensive agents that have similar cardiovascular benefits in all forms of cardiovascular disease. Other features of both ARB and ACE-I therapy are the renal-protective influence, particularly among patients who have type II diabetes and evidence of albuminuria [11]. The degree of albuminuria is reduced, and the progression to end-stage renal disease is reduced among patients who have type II diabetes. Furthermore, use of either ARB or ACE-I is linked to a decreased incidence of developing type II diabetes [12].

The mechanism of action of the ARB is different from that of ACE-I, in that the angiotensin (AT1) receptor is actually competitively inhibited by the ARB, thus preventing the well-known phenomenon of ACE-I escape [13]. Simply blocking the ACE-I does prevent the production of angiotensin II from chymase or other non–ACE-I-dependent pathways. Over time one can see a demonstrable increase in angiotensin II production, even in patients receiving ACE-I

therapy. Use of ARB blocks the receptor to all angiotensin II.

The efficacy of ARB was demonstrated first in patients who had left ventricular dysfunction in the Effect of Losartan in The Elderly (ELITE II) trial [14]. In this trial, 3152 elderly patients who had systolic heart failure were assigned randomly to either losartan titrated to 50 mg/d or captopril titrated to 50 mg three times daily. There were no significant differences in any clinical indicators of heart failure between the two groups, but losartan was better tolerated. Several other investigations using other drugs from the ARB class also have demonstrated comparable clinical efficacy of ACE-I and ARB in patients who have left ventricular dysfunction (see Box 1). In patients who have left ventricular dysfunction and develop ACE-I cough, ARB is first-line therapy.

Given the efficacy of both ACE-I therapy and ARB in left ventricular dysfunction, a logical next question was whether the addition of an ARB to standard heart failure therapy would reduce morbidity and mortality. The Valsartan Heart Failure Trial (Val-HeFT) evaluated the long-term effects of the addition of the ARB valsartan to standard therapy for heart failure [15]. A total of 5010 patients who had heart failure were assigned randomly to receive 160 mg of valsartan or placebo twice daily. The primary outcomes were mortality and the combined end point of mortality and morbidity, defined as the incidence of cardiac arrest with resuscitation, hospitalization for heart failure, or receipt of intravenous inotropic or vasodilator therapy. There was no significant difference in total mortality between the valsartan and placebo groups, but the combined end point of mortality and morbidity was reduced significantly among patients receiving valsartan as compared with those receiving placebo ($P = .009$). Although this finding was quite compelling, some concern was raised because the patients who were receiving triple therapy (ACE-I plus ARB plus beta-blocker) actually had a trend toward worse mortality and morbidity. This finding was somewhat nebulous, because fewer than 35% of the patients in the trial were receiving beta-blocker therapy.

Fortunately the concerns regarding the addition of ARB were addressed better in the prospective Candesartan in Heart Failure: Assessment of Reduction in Mortality and Morbidity (CHARM)-Added trial, part of the CHARM Program [16]. The investigators evaluated whether combining the ARB, candesartan, with ACE-I inhibitors would improve clinical outcomes. The primary outcome was cardiovascular death or unplanned admission to hospital for the management of worsening congestive heart failure. A total of 2548 patients were assigned randomly to placebo or candesartan. All patients had symptomatic left ventricular dysfunction with a mean ejection fraction of 28%; 55% of the patients used beta-blockers. Significantly fewer of the patients treated with candesartan (38%) than patients receiving placebo (42%) reached the primary end point ($P = 0.011$). In both groups, 62% of the patients had ischemia as the cause of left ventricular dysfunction. Despite the higher penetrance of beta-blocker use, there was no signal of worsening heart failure as a result of triple therapy. Furthermore, the high incidence of ischemic heart disease would seem to support the use of ARB among patients after infarction.

Given the similar clinical benefits noted in patients who have chronic heart failure, it would stand to reason that the ARBs also would be of clinical benefit for patients who have myocardial infarction and left ventricular dysfunction. The Valsartan in Acute Myocardial Infarction (VALIANT) trial was designed to test the hypothesis that treatment with valsartan, an ARB, alone or in combination with captopril, an ACE-I, would result in better survival than treatment with a proven ACE-I-inhibitor regimen [17]. The design also specified analyses to assess non-inferiority if valsartan was neither clearly superior nor clearly inferior to captopril. In VALIANT 14,703 patients receiving conventional therapy were assigned randomly, 0.5 to 10 days after acute myocardial infarction, to additional therapy with valsartan (4909 patients), valsartan plus captopril (4885 patients), or captopril (4909 patients). The primary end point was death from any cause. All the patients had left ventricular dysfunction with a left ventricular ejection fraction below 35% on echocardiography or below 40% on contrast angiography/or radionuclide ventriculography. The median follow-up was 24.7 months. There was no difference in total mortality or in combined cardiovascular end points of recurrent myocardial infarction, hospitalization for heart failure, resuscitation from cardiac arrest, and stroke.

Summary

The utilization of angiotensin-II attenuating agents is the standard of care in the management of patients with left ventricular dysfunction regardless of the etiology. The most effective agents

of this group include both angiotensin converting enzyme inhibitors and angiotensin receptor antagonists. Given the worse outcomes noted in those patients with coronary artery disease, efforts to optimize appropriate pharmacotherapy in this population is imperative. There does appear to be some advantage in the combination of ACE-I+ARB in chronic left ventricular dysfunction patients. In those patients that have sustained a recent myocardial infarction with concomitant left ventricular dysfunction, the combination of ACE-I+ARB does not improve survival and in fact might exacerbate renal dysfunction as well as hypotension. The appropriate employment of agents that attenuate the effects of angiotensin-II should be a priority in the care and management of the left ventricular dysfunction patient.

References

[1] Mann D. Inflammatory mediators and the failing heart: past, present and the foreseeable future. Circ Res 2002;91:988–98.
[2] The CONSENSUS Trial Study Group. Effects of enalapril on mortality in severe congestive heart failure. Results of the Cooperative North Scandinavian Enalapril Survival Study (CONSENSUS). N Engl J Med 1987;316(23):1429–35.
[3] Domanski M, Exner D, Borkowf C, et al. Effect of angiotensin converting enzyme inhibition on sudden cardiac death in patients following acute myocardial infarction: a meta-analysis of randomized clinical trials. J Am Coll Cardiol 1999;33(3):598–604.
[4] Pfeffer M, Braunwald E, Moye L, et al. Effect of captopril on mortality and morbidity in patients with left ventricular dysfunction after myocardial infarction. Results of the survival and ventricular enlargement trial. The SAVE Investigators. N Engl J Med 1992; 327(10):669–77.
[5] Swedberg K, Held P, Kjekshus J, et al. Effects of the early administration of enalapril on mortality in patients with acute myocardial infarction. Results of the Cooperative New Scandinavian Enalapril Survival Study II (CONSENSUS II). N Engl J Med 1992;327(23):678–84.
[6] Kober L, Torp-Petersen C, Carlsen J, et al. A clinical trial of the angiotensin-converting-enzyme inhibitor trandolapril in patients with left ventricular dysfunction after myocardial infarction TRACE Study Group. N Engl J Med 1995;333(25):1670–6.
[7] The Acute Infarction Ramipril Efficacy (AIRE) Study Investigators. Effect of ramipril on mortality and morbidity of survivors of acute myocardial infarction with clinical evidence of heart failure. Lancet 1993;342:821–8.
[8] Borghi C, Ambrosioni E, on behalf of the Survival of Myocardial Infarction Long-term Evaluation

(SMILE) Study Group. Effects of zofenopril on myocardial ischemia in post-myocardial infarction patient with preserved left ventricular function: the Survival of Myocardial Infarction Long-Term Evaluation (SMILE)–ISCHEMIA study. Am Heart J 2007;153(3):445.e7–445.e14.

[9] The European Trial on Reduction of Cardiac Events with Perindopril in Stable Coronary Artery Disease Investigators. Efficacy of perindopril in reduction of cardiovascular events among patients with stable coronary artery disease: randomized, double-blind, placebo-controlled, multicentre trial (the EUROPA study). Lancet 2003;362:782–8.

[10] Dicpinigaitis P. Angiotensin-converting enzyme inhibitor-induced cough: ACCP evidence-based clinical practice guidelines. Chest 2006;supplement 129: 169–73.

[11] Barnett A, Bain S, Bouter P, et al, Diabetics Exposed to Telmisartan and Enalapril Study Group. Angiotensin-receptor blockade versus converting-enzyme inhibition in type 2 diabetes and nephropathy. N Engl J Med 2004;351:1952–61.

[12] The ALLHAT Officers and Coordinators. Major outcomes in high-risk hypertensive patients randomized to angiotensin-converting enzyme inhibitor or calcium channel blocker vs diuretic. The Antihypertensive and Lipid-Lowering Treatment to Prevent Heart Attack Trial (ALLHAT). JAMA 2002; 288(23):2981–97.

[13] Jorde U. Suppression of the renin-angiotensin-aldosterone system in chronic heart failure: choice of agents and clinical impact. Cardiol Rev 2006;14: 81–7.

[14] Pitt B, Poole-Wilson P, Segal R, et al, On behalf of the ELITE II Investigators. Effect of losartan compared with captopril on mortality in patients with symptomatic heart failure: randomized trial—the Losartan Heart Failure Survival Study ELITE II. Lancet 2000;355:1582–7.

[15] Cohn J, Tognoni G, Bourge R, et al, for the Valsartan Heart Failure Trial Investigators. A randomized trial of the angiotensin-receptor blocker valsartan in chronic heart failure. N Engl J Med 2001;245(23): 1667–75.

[16] McMurray J, Ostergren J, Svedberg K, et al, for the CHARM Investigators and Committees. Effects of candesartan in patients with chronic heart failure and reduced left-ventricular systolic function taking angiotensin-converting-enzyme inhibitors: the CHARM-added trial. Lancet 2003;362:767–71.

[17] Pfeffer M, McMurray J, Velazquez E, et al. Valsartan, captopril, or both in myocardial infarction complicated by heart failure, left ventricular dysfunction, or both. N Engl J Med 2003;349(20): 1893–906.

[18] The SOLVD Investigators. Effect of enalapril on survival in patients with reduced left ventricular ejection fractions and congestive heart failure. N Engl J Med 1991;325(5):293–302.

[19] The SOLVD Investigators. Effect of enalapril on mortality and the development of heart failure in asymptomatic patients with reduced left ventricular ejection fractions. N Engl J Med 1992;327(10): 685–91.

[20] Pitt B, Zannad F, Remme WJ, et al. The effect of spironolactone on morbidity and mortality in patients with severe heart failure. The Randomized Aldactone Evaluation Study Investigators. N Engl J Med 1999;341(10):709–17.

[21] Yusuf S, Sleight P, Pogue J, et al. Effects of an angiotensin-converting-enzyme inhibitor, ramipril, on cardiovascular events in high-risk patients. Heart Outcomes Prevention Evaluation Study Investigators. N Engl J Med 2000;342(3):145–53.

Comprehensive Adrenergic Blockade Post Myocardial Infarction Left Ventricular Dysfunction

Gregg C. Fonarow, MD

Geffen School of Medicine at UCLA, UCLA Medical Center, Los Angeles, CA, USA

More than 1.2 million patients sustain a myocardial infarction (MI) in the United States each year [1]. Despite significant advances in pharmacologic and interventional therapies, 25% of men and 38% of women die within 1 year of an acute MI [1]. In addition, nearly half will experience subsequent physical disability from heart failure (HF) [1]. The prognosis after an MI is determined by several factors, including the extent of left ventricular systolic dysfunction (LVD) (left ventricular ejection fraction [LVEF] ≤40%) with or without clinical HF, the presence of myocardial ischemia, the extent and progression of underlying coronary artery disease, patient age, and various comorbidities. These factors lead to death due to progressive HF, sudden arrhythmic death, and reinfarction. The presence of clinical HF is associated with significantly reduced survival rates even many months after the acute event, and a low LVEF is the single most potent predictor of sudden arrhythmic death in post-MI survivors [2].

Randomized clinical trials have shown that long-term beta-blocker use reduces the risk of death and disability in MI survivors. The 2004 American Heart Association/American College of Cardiology (AHA/ACC) (ST elevation MI [STEMI]) guidelines give a class I, level of evidence A recommendation (procedure/treatment should be performed/administered) for the in-hospital and long-term post discharge use of beta-blockers in MI patients without contraindications [3]. The presence of hemodynamic instability or decompensated HF early in the course of STEMI should preclude the use of intravenous beta-blockade, but LVD with or without compensated HF is a strong indication for the oral use of beta-blockade before discharge from the hospital [3]. The 2002 ACC/AHA guideline update for the management of patients with unstable angina and non–ST segment elevation MI supports the use of beta-blocker therapy as a class I, level of evidence B recommendation [4].

Despite compelling evidence and recommendations, beta-blockers remain an underused therapy in the post-MI period. Physician concerns may exist regarding the safety and benefits of beta-blockers in post-MI patients with LVD, with or without HF symptoms, despite clinical trial evidence to the contrary. Many post-MI patients have LVD even in the absence of symptoms of HF. In the Trandolapril Cardiac Evaluation (TRACE) registry involving more than 6500 post-MI patients, the presence of HF and LVD were assessed within the first few days after presentation. This study found that 64% of post-MI patients had either HF or LVD or both [5,6]. Misunderstandings may also persist regarding the safety and benefits of beta-blockers in elderly patients or patients with diabetes or chronic obstructive airway disease post MI. Several beta-blockers have demonstrated safety and efficacy in large-scale, long-term, placebo-controlled, randomized clinical trials of MI survivors in which the target doses were well defined [7–9]. Nevertheless, MI patients are often treated with agents whose long-term use has not been shown to be effective and for which optimal dosing has not been defined [10,11].

E-mail address: gfonarow@mednet.ucla.edu

0733-8651/08/$ - see front matter © 2008 Elsevier Inc. All rights reserved.
doi:10.1016/j.ccl.2007.08.006

Post myocardial infarction and left ventricular dysfunction: a dangerous intersection

Many studies have demonstrated that patients presenting with LVD with or without clinical HF post MI are at higher risk for adverse outcomes, including cardiac rupture, cardiac arrest, stroke, longer hospitalizations, ventricular arrhythmias, recurrent MI, and death [12–14]. Within 6 years of a MI, approximately 18% of men and 35% of women will have a recurrent MI. Post-MI patients also have a sudden death rate that is four to six times that of the general population [3]. When compared with post-MI patients without LVD, patients with LVD have an even worse prognosis. Post-MI patients with LVD have a fourfold increase in the rate of in-hospital mortality and a two- to threefold increase in the rate of mortality at 30 days and 6 months [12–14]. Data from the Global Registry of Acute Coronary Events (GRACE) study demonstrated that patients with acute coronary syndromes who presented with HF on admission were at increased risk of in-hospital mortality (12.0% versus 2.9% without HF; $P < .0001$) and 6-month mortality (8.5% versus 2.8% without HF; $P < .0001$) [14]. Post-MI patients with LVD also have a twofold increase in the rate of reinfarction. Approximately 50% of patients with LVD do not have symptoms of HF, but despite being asymptomatic, they remain at similar risk as patients with symptoms of HF [15].

Post-MI patients with LVD and HF are at high risk to die unexpectedly. Patients with LVD without HF symptoms are also at high risk for sudden death. An analysis of data from the Valsartan in Acute Myocardial Infarction Trial (VALIANT) assessed the incidence and timing of sudden unexpected death in post-MI patients with LVD [2]. Of 14,609 patients, 1067 (7%) had an event after MI; 903 died suddenly and 164 were resuscitated after cardiac arrest [2]. Of the 3852 patients with an LVEF of 30% or less, 10% died suddenly or had cardiac arrest with resuscitation during the trial as compared with 6% of the 4998 patients with an LVEF of 31% to 40% and 5% of the 2406 patients with an LVEF of more than 40%. The event risk was highest (1.4%) in the first 30 days after MI and decreased to 0.14% per month after 2 years [2]. The rate of sudden death according to LVEF showed that the increased early incidence was most apparent among patients with low LVEF; of the sudden deaths that occurred during the first 30 days,

54% occurred among the patients with an LVEF of 30% or less [2].

The absence of HF symptoms in post-MI patients, especially in those who have undergone thrombolysis, percutaneous coronary interventions, or coronary artery bypass grafting surgery may result in unrecognized LVD, depriving patients of therapies that can prevent future HF and reduce the risk of death, arrhythmias, reinfarction, and sudden death. Measurement of LVEF post MI is extremely important due to the large increase in risk associated with the diagnosis of LVD [3].

Neurohormonal blockade post myocardial infarction

Activation of the sympathetic nervous system and the renin-angiotensin-aldosterone system (RAAS) has been associated with left ventricular remodeling, worsening HF, recurrent ischemic events, arrhythmias, and mortality in MI survivors [16]. Myocardial injury and ventricular dysfunction lead to a baroreceptor-mediated increase in sympathetic tone. This activation results in an increase in myocardial contractility and systemic vasoconstriction (arterial and venous) and increased myocardial oxygen consumption, cardiac afterload, and cardiac preload. Activation of the sympathetic nervous system is characterized by increased plasma levels of catecholamines (eg, epinephrine and norepinephrine). The deleterious effects of epinephrine and norepinephrine on the heart and circulation include cardiac myocyte death and dysfunction, increased ventricular size and pressures, proarrhythmic effects, and increased heart rate (Fig. 1) [6]. Although the beta-1 adrenergic receptor is the most prevalent receptor in the normal heart, post-MI and HF myocardial cells express higher proportions of beta-2 and alpha-1 adrenergic receptors, and events mediated through these receptors increase in importance in the post-MI heart with LVD. Increased local and circulating concentrations of norepinephrine contribute to myocyte hypertrophy directly through stimulation of alpha-1, beta-1, and beta-2 adrenergic receptors and indirectly via activation of the RAAS. Norepinephrine has also been shown to be toxic to myocardial cells through calcium overload (necrosis) and induction of apoptosis. Adrenergic stimulation also induces myocardial proinflammatory cytokine production. Higher levels of circulating

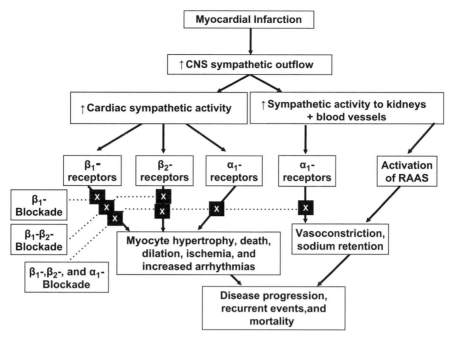

Fig. 1. Sympathetic nervous system activation and disease progression after MI. With development of MI and LVD, chronic activation of the sympathetic adrenergic system is toxic to the heart and contributes to disease progression. Three adrenergic receptors on human cardiac myocytes produce deleterious effects: β_1, β_2, and α_1. Large trials of adrenergic receptor antagonists have proved that inhibiting adrenergic stimulation is effective for reduction of cardiac morbidity and mortality in patients post MI. CNS, central nervous system.

plasma norepinephrine correlate with a poorer long-term prognosis.

Pharmacologic inhibition of these neurohormonal pathways has been evaluated in a large number of randomized post-MI clinical trials [3,4,6,16]. Certain beta-blockers, angiotensin-converting enzyme (ACE) inhibitors, and angiotensin receptor antagonists have been demonstrated to significantly reduce post-MI mortality and morbidity and are now included in clinical guideline recommendations as standards of care [3]. The use of these agents leads to clinical benefits such as reduced ischemia, reinfarction, HF, sudden death, and mortality. Evidence suggests that more comprehensive adrenergic blockade provides additional benefit in the treatment of LVD and HF post MI when compared with blockade of only the beta-1 adrenergic receptor. Because stimulation of all three adrenergic receptors may be involved in promoting myocardial toxicity, medications providing more comprehensive adrenergic blockade counteract increased sympathetic activity more completely than selective beta antagonists.

Efficacy of beta-blockers after myocardial infarction

Early post myocardial infarction period

Oral beta-blocker use in the immediate (first 24 hours) post-MI period is a class I, level of evidence A recommendation in the AHA/ACC guidelines [3]. The use of intravenous beta-blockers in patients without contraindications such as hypotension or decompensated HF is a class IIA, level of evidence B recommendation [3]. Some, but not all, trials of beta-blockers in the early stage after an MI have shown a reduced risk of reinfarction, arrhythmias, and mortality [16]. Beta-blockers are believed to limit the damage to the injured myocardium [17]. Prior meta-analyses of clinical trials have demonstrated that early (within 24 hours) post-MI beta-blocker use can provide reductions in all-cause mortality; however, there was less clear evidence of a reduction in nonfatal reinfarction [10,18–21]. These trials generally excluded patients with HF or LVD. Most of these intravenous followed by oral beta-blocker trials were conducted before the use of reperfusion therapy and other standard of care therapies for MI [20].

The large-scale Clopidogrel and Metoprolol in Myocardial Infarction Trial (COMMIT) showed no mortality difference with the use of intravenous followed by short-term oral beta-1 selective blockade [22]. In that study, 45,852 patients were randomly allocated to metoprolol therapy (up to 15 mg of intravenous metoprolol tartrate, then 200 mg orally of daily metoprolol succinate; n = 22,929) or matching placebo (n = 22,923). Study treatment was to continue until discharge or up to 4 weeks in hospital (mean, 15 days). Eligible patients included those presenting with ST-segment elevation, left bundle branch block, or ST-segment depression (7%) within 24 hours of the onset of symptoms of suspected acute MI, unless their physician considered them to have clear indications for, or contraindications to, any of the study treatments. Patients scheduled for primary percutaneous coronary intervention were excluded. Other reasons for excluding patients were determined by the physician and included either a small likelihood of worthwhile benefit (eg, other life-threatening disease or an unconvincing history of MI) or a high risk of adverse effects with the study treatments (including persistently low blood pressure [eg, systolic blood pressure below 100 mm Hg], low heart rate [eg, below 50 bpm], heart block, or cardiogenic shock). Evidence of moderate HF (Killip class II or III) was not an exclusion criterion; approximately 20% of patients were in Killip class II and almost 5% were classified as Killip class III. The trial demonstrated that there was no difference in overall mortality between the placebo and metoprolol groups (relative risk [RR] = 1%, P = .7). Importantly, patients in this study had a significantly increased risk (30%, P < .00001) of cardiogenic shock when administered intravenous metoprolol tartrate followed by oral metoprolol succinate versus placebo, which was observed consistently across all categories of patients [22]. In higher-risk patients, for the combined safety and efficacy outcome, allocation to metoprolol resulted in a marked increase in risk (absolute increase of 43.7 ± 13.0 per 1000 patients treated). Consequently, the early safety and efficacy of using intravenous beta-blocker therapy in post-MI patients has been questioned.

Intermediate and long-term post–myocardial infarction period

Long-term beta-blocker therapy has been associated with significant mortality reductions in

MI patients as demonstrated in three large-scale, randomized, clinical trials—the Beta-Blocker Heart Attack Trial (BHAT), [7,23] the Norwegian Timolol Trial (NTT), [8] and the Carvedilol Post-Infarct Survival Control in Left Ventricular Dysfunction (CAPRICORN) [9] trial (Table 1) [24]. Notably, these trials demonstrating benefit post MI all used nonselective beta-blockers. The one large-scale, longer-term trial of a selective beta-blocker post MI, the Lopressor Intervention Trial (LIT), failed to demonstrated a reduction in the risk of mortality or recurrent infarction in a comparison with placebo (Table 1).

Although HF or LVD is present in a large number of MI patients, [6] individuals with significant cardiac decompensation have generally been excluded from randomized beta-blocker trials. Only 19% of BHAT and 33% of NTT participants had a history or some degree of HF on admission [8,23]. In BHAT, patients with a history of severe HF were excluded, and in NTT, patients with uncontrolled cardiac failure were excluded [7,8]. CAPRICORN specifically enlisted only patients with documented LVD and was performed in the era of thrombolysis, angioplasty, and ACE inhibitor therapy [9]. Patients were randomized to carvedilol as early as the day following the infarct, and the majority were randomized within the first 2 weeks of the trial. CAPRICORN demonstrated that when carvedilol was added to standard care (including antiplatelet therapy, ACE inhibitors, lipid-lowering and, if indicated, reperfusion therapy) and compared with placebo added to standard care, there was a statistically significant 23% reduction in all-cause mortality (Fig. 2) [9]. CAPRICORN further demonstrated that carvedilol reduced the risk of reinfarction by 40% [25,26]. Half of the patients in CAPRICORN had no current or prior HF symptoms (asymptomatic, stage B), and 46% were given acute interventional therapy (either thrombolytic therapy or angioplasty) [9]. Carvedilol resulted in similar benefit in patients with no symptoms of HF (RR = 31%) and in those who had undergone revascularization (RR = 32%) [25]. In a subgroup analysis, carvedilol also significantly increased the LVEF, whereas placebo caused no change after 6 months of treatment [27].

Evidence-based strategy for post–myocardial infarction beta-blocker therapy

A meta-analysis of post-MI trials suggested that beta-1-selective blockers had a lesser

Table 1
Large trials of oral beta-blockers in acute/post MI

Study	Length of trial	Active treatment	Beta-blocker	Number of patients	Background therapy	Mortality	Fatal/nonfatal reinfarction	Assessed HF/LVD
Goteborg [18]	3 mo	Metoprolol[a]	Selective (β₁)	1395	None	↓36%, P = .024	P = NS	Excluded HF
BHAT [7,23]	25 mo	Propranolol	Nonselective (β₁, β₂)	3837	No acute therapies; ACEI = none reported or not available; lipid-lowering agents (3%), aspirin (21%)	↓26%, P <.005	P = NS	Excluded HF
NTT [8]	17 mo	Timolol	Nonselective (β₁, β₂)	1884	ACEI, aspirin = none reported; lipid-lowering agents = not available	↓39%, P = .003	↓28%, P = .0005	Excluded HF
LIT [11]	12 mo	Metoprolol	Selective (β₁)	2395	ACEI = none reported; lipid-lowering agents = not available; aspirin = excluded	↑4%, P = NS	P = NS	Excluded HF
CAPRICORN [9,24]	15 mo	Carvedilol	Nonselective (β₁, β₂, α₁)	1959	Acute: IV nitrates (73%), heparin (64%), thrombolytics (37%), diuretics (34%) Long term: ACEI (98%), aspirin (86%), statins (23%), reperfusion therapy (46%)	↓23, P = .031	↓40, P = .01	Included acute LVD and HF

Abbreviations: ACEI, angiotensin-converting enzyme inhibitors; CHF, congestive heart failure; Goteborg, Goteborg Metoprolol Trial; IV, intravenous; NA, not available; NS, not significant.

[a] Patients received IV (15 mg) followed by oral metoprolol tartrate (200 mg).

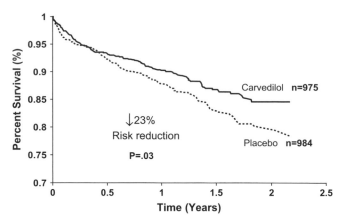

Fig. 2. Effect of carvedilol in post-MI patients with LVD. In the CAPRICORN study, carvedilol treatment after an MI significantly reduced the risk of mortality when compared with placebo. (*From* CAPRICORN Investigators. Effect of carvedilol on outcome after myocardial infarction in patients with left-ventricular dysfunction: the CAPRICORN randomized trial. Lancet 2001;357:1387; with permission.)

mortality benefit in acute MI survivors when compared with beta-blockers with beta-2- or alpha-1-blocking properties [28]. This meta-analysis of 32 randomized, placebo-controlled, post-acute MI trials involving 26,580 patients revealed a greater mortality risk reduction relative to placebo using nonselective beta-blockers (carvedilol, timolol, propranolol) when compared with beta-1-selective blockers (immediate- and controlled-release metoprolol, bisoprolol, and atenolol), with mortality risk reductions of 31% and 21%, respectively [28].

Although large-scale randomized clinical trials have demonstrated a reduced post-MI mortality risk in patients with normal ventricular function treated with long-term propranolol (BHAT) [7] and timolol (NTT) [8] and in patients with LVD treated with carvedilol (CAPRICORN) [9], no similar evidence has been reported for the commonly used beta-1-selective blockers metoprolol tartrate, metoprolol succinate, or atenolol. In general, although anti-adrenergic agents are discussed as being interchangeable, the currently available clinical trial evidence does not support the view that clinical benefits of beta-blockers post MI are a class effect. More comprehensive adrenergic blockage appears to provide greater benefits. Carvedilol is unique in that it does not exhibit the carbohydrate and lipid disturbances that may underlie the apparent failure of some traditional beta-blockers to reduce cardiovascular morbidity and mortality. Traditional beta-blockers decrease insulin sensitivity and glucose utilization and increase the atherogenicity of serum lipids, whereas carvedilol has demonstrated an overall positive influence on these metabolic factors.

Evidence-based algorithm for beta-blockers post myocardial infarction

Patients with suspected myocardial infarction admitted to the hospital
Initiating intravenous beta-blockers. In MI patients with significant ongoing chest pain, hypertension, or marked sinus tachycardia without contraindications, intravenous dosing may be considered; otherwise, oral dosing should be initiated. MI patients receiving intravenous beta-blockers require strict monitoring of heart rate, blood pressure, electrocardiogram, and clinical status during initiation, and administration should be discontinued if abnormalities occur. The AHA/ACC guidelines state that intravenous beta-blocker use is a class IIA recommendation [3]. Intravenous beta-blockers should be avoided in all patients with hypotension, hemodynamic instability, or HF.

Current guidelines state that all patients should be prescribed an oral beta-blocker after an MI unless there is an absolute contraindication to therapy. Contraindications include symptomatic bradycardia, hypotension (systolic blood pressure <80 mm Hg), signs of peripheral hypoperfusion, cardiogenic shock, acute pulmonary edema, advanced heart block (without pacemaker), or reactive airway disease [3].

Many patients are initiated intravenously on beta-1-selective agents in hospital, converted to oral treatment, and discharged on these beta-1-selective agents despite their failure to demonstrate significant improvement in long-term survival after MI [10,11]. Implementation of evidence-based therapy may prompt consideration of switching patients from beta-1-selective blockers to nonselective beta-blockers. Switching was performed safely in MI patients during the CAPRICORN trial, in which prior beta-blockade did not exclude participation [9]. A post-hoc analysis including the approximately 15% of CAPRICORN patients who had received at least one dose of intravenous or oral beta-blockade was performed. The agent was discontinued before randomization. Although some of these patients were switched to carvedilol on the same day, the majority had one or more intervening days with no beta-blocker therapy. Carvedilol resulted in clinical benefits regardless of whether patients had initially been started on a different beta-blocker or were started de novo at randomization. Patients initiated on an intravenous or oral beta-blocker who subsequently received carvedilol had the same improved outcomes as those initiated directly on carvedilol [27,29].

Among patients randomized in the hospital in CAPRICORN, there was no significant heterogeneity between those newly started on or those switched to carvedilol with regard to in-hospital HF or bradycardia adverse events. Importantly, patients newly started on carvedilol had similar rates of in-hospital HF and bradycardia as those on placebo (HF: placebo 2%, carvedilol 4%, $P = .06$; bradycardia: placebo 2%, carvedilol 1%, $P = .77$). This pattern was also seen for patients who had previously received intravenous or oral beta-blockade (HF: placebo 1%, carvedilol 2%, $P = .28$; bradycardia: placebo 2%, carvedilol 3%, $P = .56$). For in-hospital hypotensive events, there was a trend toward heterogeneity between these subgroups (interaction P value $= .08$). Eleven percent of patients newly started on carvedilol experienced a hypotensive event compared with 6% on placebo ($P = .0007$); however, there were nearly equal rates (7% placebo, 8% carvedilol) among patients previously receiving intravenous or oral beta-blockade as part of their post-MI treatment [25,27,29].

No difference was observed between the carvedilol and placebo groups in the incidence of HF adverse events reported any time during the study regardless of prior beta-blocker treatment. For bradycardia, patients newly started on carvedilol had a rate of 7.5% any time during the study versus 4% for placebo ($P = .0005$); for patients who previously received a beta-blocker, this rate was 8% for carvedilol and 5% for placebo ($P = .06$). For hypotension any time during the study, patients newly started on carvedilol had a rate of 24% versus 15% on placebo ($P < .0001$); for patients who previously received beta-blockade, this rate was 21% on carvedilol versus 14% on placebo ($P = .03$) [25,27,29].

Withdrawal of medication, for events in-hospital and for events reported for the entire study, showed no heterogeneity based on prior beta-blocker use and no difference between carvedilol and placebo [29]. Although these data primarily reflect a population that was not directly switched from intravenous or oral beta-blocker therapy to carvedilol in the peri-MI period, they suggest the safety and efficacy of carvedilol in such patients [27].

Initiating oral beta-blockers. Oral beta-blockers may be started before, during, or after initiation and titration of ACE inhibitor or angiotensin receptor blocker (ARB) therapy in patients with or without reperfusion therapy [3]. The evidence-based beta-blockers for post-MI patients without LVD include propranolol and timolol (Table 2). Both metoprolol tartrate and atenolol are indicated for post-MI use by the US Food and Drug Administration (FDA), although their safety and efficacy, specifically in post-MI patients with LVD, has not been studied. Evidence from CAPRICORN shows that patients with LVD, regardless of the presence of HF symptoms, benefit greatly from treatment [9,25]. Left ventricular function should be assessed in the hospital before the patient is discharged, and an LVEF less than or equal to 40% warrants the use of carvedilol preferentially. Carvedilol is the only beta-blocker that is FDA approved in patients post MI with LVD [25]. A new once-a-day formulation of carvedilol (carvedilol controlled release) was approved by the FDA in October 2006 for all of the same indications as carvedilol twice daily: mild-to-severe HF, post-MI LVD with or without symptoms of HF, and hypertension. Studies have shown that carvedilol twice daily and carvedilol controlled release are bioequivalent [25].

In patients with LVD, carvedilol should be started at 6.25 mg twice daily and increased to 12.5 and 25 mg twice daily at 3- to 10-day intervals (Table 3) [9,25]. The recommended dosing regimen need not be altered in patients who received treatment with an intravenous or oral

Table 2

Recommended dosing for evidence-based beta-blockers in post-MI patients

No LVD or HF[a]

Agent	Initiation dose	Target dose
Timolol	5 mg bid	10 mg bid
Propranolol	40 mg qid	60 to 80 mg qid

LVD with or without HF[b]

Agent	Initiation dose	Titration steps (3–10 days after initiation)	Target dose
Carvedilol	6.25 mg bid[c]	12.5 mg bid	25 mg bid
Carvedilol CR	20 mg qd	40 mg qd	80 mg qd

[a] *Data from* Refs. [7,8].

[b] *Data from* Refs. [9,25].

[c] A lower starting dose may be used (3.125 mg twice daily or 10 mg once daily), or the rate of up titration may be slowed if clinically indicated (eg, due to low blood pressure, low heart rate, or fluid retention). Patients should be maintained on lower doses if higher doses are not tolerated.

beta-blocker during the acute phase of the MI. Treatment should be initiated as soon as possible, and the target dose should be continued indefinitely. If patients are unable to achieve the full recommended dose due to severe bradycardia or hypotension, a lower dose should be maintained and dose escalation should be reattempted after several weeks. Dose-related clinical benefits have been demonstrated at below target doses of carvedilol in patients with chronic HF [30].

Table 3

American College of Cardiology/American Heart Association guidelines for management of ST elevation MI

Acute therapy	Discharge therapy
Aspirin	Aspirin
Clopidogrel	Clopidogrel
Beta-blocker	Beta-blocker
Heparin (UFH or LMWH)	ACE inhibitor/ARB
GP IIb-IIIa inhibitor (if receiving PCI)	Aldosterone antagonist if LVD
Cath/PCI	Statin/lipid-lowering drug
Reperfusion	Smoking cessation
	Cardiac rehabilitation

Abbreviations: Cath, catheterization; GP, glycoprotein; LMHW, low-molecular-weight heparin; PCI, percutaneous coronary intervention; UFH, unfractionated heparin.

Data from Antman EM, Anbe DT, Armstrong PW, et al. ACC/AHA guidelines for the management of patients with ST-elevation myocardial infarction executive summary: a report of the American College of Cardiology/American Heart Association Task Force on Practice Guidelines (Writing Committee to Revise the 1999 Guidelines for the Management of Patients With Acute Myocardial Infarction). Circulation 2004;110:588–636.

Concomitant drug therapy

The ACC/AHA recommendations for pharmacologic therapy in the acute phase after MI and long-term management are listed in Table 3. Patients with MI should be treated with ACE inhibitors and beta-blockers in the absence of contraindications, irrespective of left ventricular function [3]. In post-MI patients with LVD and HF, aldosterone antagonists are also indicated in the absence of contraindications or intolerance [3]. ACE inhibitors are class I recommended in higher-risk patients for initiation 12 to 24 hours after admission for MI; therefore, patients may be started on beta-blockers before, during, or after initiation of ACE inhibitors. ACE inhibitors do not need to be at target doses before the initiation of a beta-blocker. Subsequent up titration of the ACE inhibitor can be done after optimization of the beta-blocker dose, and both agents may be titrated to target doses over time. Aldosterone antagonists are recommended in post-MI patients with LVD, HF, or diabetes in the absence of contraindications or significant renal dysfunction [3]. Patients must be closely monitored for the development of hyperkalemia. Aldosterone antagonists can be initiated, continued, or dose adjusted before or during beta-blocker treatment. Although both ACE inhibitors and beta-blockers are class I recommendations in the guidelines and although the evidence is strong that both should ultimately be used in post-MI patients without contraindications or intolerance [3], the question frequently arises of which to initiate first. In the major clinical trials of ACE inhibitors in MI, most patients were already on beta-blocker therapy when randomized to ACE inhibitor or placebo. In CAPRICORN, by study design, patients needed to be on ACE inhibitor therapy before randomization to carvedilol or placebo. The recent CIBIS III trial indicates that the initiation of bisoprolol before enalapril in HF may result in better outcomes for the patient [31].

In a recent clinical trial, HF patients were randomized to initiation and up titration of ACE inhibitor therapy followed by carvedilol compared with initiation and uptitration of carvedilol followed by ACE inhibitor [32]. Patients started first on carvedilol had a better clinical status, greater LVEF, and lower B-type natriuretic peptide levels at the end of 1 year when compared with those started on ACE inhibitors first. In post-MI patients with LVD and borderline blood pressures, initiation of beta-blocker therapy first followed by subsequent initiation of ACE inhibitors should be considered.

If overt HF develops in patients with asymptomatic LVD or worsens in those who already have signs or symptoms of decompensation, diuretics should be increased, and the rate of up titration should be slowed. If hypotension limits carvedilol up titration, the ACE inhibitor dose should be decreased temporarily.

Implementation of beta-blocker therapy post myocardial infarction

Despite compelling evidence of their efficacy, beta-blockers are still significantly underused in the acute setting, at discharge, and at post discharge, creating a large burden of preventable mortality, reinfarction, and HF. The Second National Registry of Myocardial Infarction compiled acute MI data from 1674 participating hospitals throughout the United States from 1994 to 1998 [12,33]. In 190,518 acute MI hospital admissions, oral beta-blockers were given at discharge to 48% of patients with HF and to 42% of those without HF [12,33]. Recent 2004 data from the Global Registry of Acute Coronary Events (GRACE) identified 1778 patients with an admission diagnosis of HF (Killip class II or III) from a pool of 94 hospitals. Patients who had HF on initial evaluation were less likely to receive beta-blockers than those diagnosed with HF in the hospital (70% versus 76%, respectively) [14]. An investigation into recent changes in the quality of care delivered to Medicare beneficiaries found that 64% of MI patients considered ideal candidates were treated with beta-blocker therapy within 24 hours and 72% were on beta-blocker

therapy at discharge in the years 1998 to 1999. The data from 2000 to 2001 showed a modest improvement, with 69% and 79% of ideal MI patients taking beta-blocker therapy within 24 hours and upon discharge, respectively [34].

ACC/AHA performance measures for MI include measures for the use of beta-blockers in the first 24 hours and at discharge for eligible patients without contraindications or intolerance. Numerous studies have demonstrated the role of hospital-based systems in improving quality of care; moreover, such programs are substantially more effective than usual care. Outpatient disease management, preventive cardiology programs, and cardiac rehabilitation programs can improve treatment rates and patient adherence to therapy. The AHA and ACC recommend the use of programs such as the "AHA's Get With The Guidelines" or the "ACC's Guidelines Applied to Practice" to identify appropriate patients for therapy, to provide practitioners with useful reminders based on the guidelines, and to continuously assess the success achieved in providing these therapies to the patients who can benefit from them [3].

Summary

A convincing body of evidence supports the lifesaving benefits of beta-blocker therapy in post-MI patients. Based on this evidence, the latest ACC/AHA guidelines for MI indicate that all patients without contraindications should be started on beta-blocker therapy, irrespective of concomitant fibrinolytic therapy or the performance of primary percutaneous coronary intervention [3]. There is little evidence that a class effect exists, and attempts should be made to use the specific agents and doses demonstrated to be effective in randomized clinical trials. Despite the results of clinical trials and national guidelines, evidence-based therapies continue to be underused in conventional practice settings. Every effort should be made to ensure that each and every eligible patient is treated with these evidence-based, guideline-recommended, life-prolonging therapies in the absence of contraindications or intolerance.

References

[1] American Heart Association. Heart disease and stroke statistics—2007 update. Dallas (TX): American Heart Association; 2007.
[2] Solomon SD, Zelenkofske S, McMurray JJ, et al. Sudden death in patients with myocardial infarction

and left ventricular dysfunction, heart failure, or both. N Engl J Med 2005;352(25):2581–8.

[3] Antman EM, Anbe DT, Armstrong PW, et al. ACC/AHA guidelines for the management of patients with ST-elevation myocardial infarction—executive summary: a report of the American College of Cardiology/American Heart Association Task Force on Practice Guidelines (Writing Committee to Revise the 1999 Guidelines for the Management of Patients With Acute Myocardial Infarction). Circulation 2004;110:588–636.

[4] Braunwald E, Antman EM, Beasley JW, et al. ACC/AHA guideline update for the management of patients with unstable angina and non-ST-segment elevation myocardial infarction: a report of the American College of Cardiology/American Heart Association Task Force on Practice Guidelines (Committee on the Management of Patients with Unstable Angina). Available at: http://www.acc.org/clinical/guidelines/unstable/unstable.pdf. Accessed: March 16, 2007.

[5] Kober L, Torp-Pedersen C, Carlsen JE, et al. A clinical trial of the angiotensin-converting-enzyme inhibitor trandolapril in patients with left ventricular dysfunction after myocardial infarction: Trandolapril Cardiac Evaluation (TRACE) Study Group. N Engl J Med 1995;333:1670–6.

[6] Cleland JG, Torabi A, Khan NK. Epidemiology and management of heart failure and left ventricular systolic dysfunction in the aftermath of a myocardial infarction. Heart 2005;91(Suppl 2):ii7–13.

[7] Beta-Blocker Heart Attack Trial Research Group. A randomized trial of propranolol in patients with acute myocardial infarction. I. Mortality results. JAMA 1982;247:1707–14.

[8] Norwegian Multicenter Study Group. Timolol-induced reduction in mortality and reinfarction in patients surviving acute myocardial infarction. N Engl J Med 1981;304:801–7.

[9] CAPRICORN Investigators. Effect of carvedilol on outcome after myocardial infarction in patients with left-ventricular dysfunction: the CAPRICORN randomised trial. Lancet 2001;357:1385–90.

[10] ISIS-1 Collaborative Group. Randomised trial of intravenous atenolol among 16,027 cases of suspected acute myocardial infarction: ISIS-1. First International Study of Infarct Survival Collaborative Group. Lancet 1986;2:57–66.

[11] Lopressor Intervention Trial Research Group. The Lopressor Intervention Trial: multicentre study of metoprolol in survivors of acute myocardial infarction. Lopressor Intervention Trial Research Group. Eur Heart J 1987;8:1056–64.

[12] Wu AH, Parsons L, Every NR, et al. Hospital outcomes in patients presenting with congestive heart failure complicating acute myocardial infarction: a report from the Second National Registry of Myocardial Infarction (NRMI-2). J Am Coll Cardiol 2002;40:1389–94.

[13] Hasdai D, Topol EJ, Kilaru R, et al. Frequency, patient characteristics, and outcomes of mild-to-moderate heart failure complicating ST-segment elevation acute myocardial infarction: lessons from 4 international fibrinolytic therapy trials. Am Heart J 2003;145:73–9.

[14] Steg PG, Dabbous OH, Feldman LJ, et al. Determinants and prognostic impact of heart failure complicating acute coronary syndromes: observations from the Global Registry of Acute Coronary Events (GRACE). Circulation 2004;109:494–9.

[15] Wang TJ, Levy D, Benjamin EJ, et al. The epidemiology of "asymptomatic" left ventricular systolic dysfunction: implications for screening. Ann Intern Med 2003;138:907–16.

[16] Weir R, McMurray JJ. Treatments that improve outcome in the patient with heart failure, left ventricular systolic dysfunction, or both after acute myocardial infarction. Heart 2005;91(Suppl 2):ii17–20.

[17] Fonarow GC. The management of the diabetic patient with prior cardiovascular events. Rev Cardiovasc Med 2003;4(Suppl 6):S38–49.

[18] Hjalmarson A, Herlitz J, Holmberg S, et al. The Goteborg metoprolol trial: effects on mortality and morbidity in acute myocardial infarction. Circulation 1983;67:I26–32.

[19] MIAMI Trial Research Group. Metoprolol in acute myocardial infarction (MIAMI): a randomised placebo-controlled international trial. The MIAMI Trial Research Group. Eur Heart J 1985;6:199–226.

[20] Freemantle N, Cleland J, Young P, et al. Beta-blockade after myocardial infarction: systematic review and meta-regression analysis. BMJ 1999;318:1730–7.

[21] Roberts R, Rogers WJ, Mueller HS, et al. Immediate versus deferred beta-blockade following thrombolytic therapy in patients with acute myocardial infarction: results of the Thrombolysis in Myocardial Infarction (TIMI) II-B Study. Circulation 1991;83:422–37.

[22] Chen ZM, Pan HC, Chen YP, et al. Early intravenous then oral metoprolol in 45,852 patients with acute myocardial infarction: randomised placebo-controlled trial. Lancet 2005;366:1622–32.

[23] Beta-Blocker Heart Attack Trial Research Group. A randomized trial of propranolol in patients with acute myocardial infarction. II. Morbidity results. JAMA 1983;250:2814–9.

[24] Sackner-Bernstein JD. New evidence from the CAPRICORN trial: the role of carvedilol in high-risk, post-myocardial infarction patients. Rev Cardiovasc Med 2003;4(Suppl 3):S25–9.

[25] COREG and COREG CR (carvedilol) tablets [prescribing information]. Research Triangle Park, NC, GlaxoSmithKline; 2006.

[26] Lopez-Sendon Hentsch J, Dargie H, Remme W, et al. Effect of carvedilol on mortality and reinfarction in left ventricular dysfunction after infarction: a subgroup analysis from CAPRICORN study. Eur Heart J 2002;4:396.

[27] Doughty RN, Whalley GA, Walsh HA, et al. Effects of carvedilol on left ventricular remodeling after acute myocardial infarction: the CAPRICORN Echo Substudy. Circulation 2004;109:201–6.

[28] Packer M. Do beta-blockers prolong survival in heart failure only by inhibiting the beta-1-receptor? A perspective on the results of the COMET trial. J Card Fail 2003;9:429–43.

[29] Fonarow GC. Practical considerations of beta-blockade in the management of the post-myocardial infarction patient. Am Heart J 2005;149:984–93.

[30] Bristow MR, Gilbert EM, Abraham WT, et al. Carvedilol produces dose-related improvements in left ventricular function and survival in subjects with chronic heart failure: MOCHA investigators. Circulation 1996;94:2807–16.

[31] Willenheimer R, van Veldhuisen DJ, Silke B, et al. Effect on survival and hospitalization of initiating treatment for chronic heart failure with bisoprolol followed by enalapril, as compared with the opposite sequence: results of the randomized Cardiac Insufficiency Bisoprolol Study (CIBIS) III. Circulation 2005;112:2426–35.

[32] Sliwa K, Norton GR, Kone N, et al. Impact of initiating carvedilol before angiotensin-converting enzyme inhibitor therapy on cardiac function in newly diagnosed heart failure. J Am Coll Cardiol 2004;44:1825–30.

[33] Becker RC, Burns M, Gore JM, et al. Early assessment and in-hospital management of patients with acute myocardial infarction at increased risk for adverse outcomes: a nationwide perspective of current clinical practice. The National Registry of Myocardial Infarction (NRMI-2) Participants. Am Heart J 1998;135:786–96.

[34] Jencks SF, Huff ED, Cuerdon T. Change in the quality of care delivered to Medicare beneficiaries, 1998–1999 to 2000–2001. JAMA 2003;289:305–12.

ELSEVIER
SAUNDERS

Cardiol Clin 26 (2008) 91–105

CARDIOLOGY
CLINICS

Aldosterone Receptor Blockade in Patients with Left Ventricular Systolic Dysfunction Following Acute Myocardial Infarction

Filippo Brandimarte, MD[a], John E.A. Blair, MD[b],
Amin Manuchehry, MD[b], Francesco Fedele, MD[a],
Mihai Gheorghiade, MD[b],*

[a]La Sapienza University, Rome, Italy
[b]Northwestern University, Feinberg School of Medicine, Chicago, IL, USA

Acute myocardial infarction (AMI) is extremely prevalent worldwide, with an estimated 700,000 new cases this year and a total mortality of 221,000 in 2002 in the United States alone [1]. Left ventricular systolic dysfunction (LVSD), as evidenced by the presence of new heart failure (HF) symptoms at the time of AMI or by documented reduction in left ventricular ejection fraction (LVEF), is common, with reported incidences of approximately 30% post-AMI [2–6]. Patients with LVSD following AMI are at high risk of in-hospital and long-term morbidity and mortality. Analysis of the Second National Registry of Myocardial Infarction (NRMI-2) demonstrated a 3-fold increase of in-hospital death (21% versus 7%) in patients hospitalized for AMI with clinical evidence of LVSD compared with those without LVSD [4]. In the Global Registry of Acute Coronary Events (GRACE), patients with clinical evidence of LVSD on admission for acute coronary syndromes (ACS) had a threefold increase in 6-month mortality (9% versus 3%) and a higher rehospitalization rate (24% versus 16%) than other patients with ACS [3].

Patients with LVSD after AMI are at a critical point in time when two different disease processes, coronary artery disease (CAD) and LVSD, are at work. The presence of underlying CAD with recent thrombosis places these patients at high risk for reinfarction, ischemia, and progression of their CAD. In addition, LVSD may progress to the development of HF, worsening pump function, ventricular arrhythmias, and sudden cardiac death (SCD). Targeting the ischemia associated with AMI, the underlying CAD, and the ventricular remodeling associated with LVSD can minimize the deleterious consequences of CAD and LVSD. Failure to attack these targets and to initiate life-saving therapies results in future morbidity and mortality.

Significant progress has been made in the development of acute reperfusion strategies, platelet inhibition, and ischemia reduction that are of critical importance in the acute phase of AMI. Secondary prevention measures for CAD, such as aspirin, clopidogrel, beta blockers, angiotensin converting enzyme (ACE) inhibitors and the use of hydroxymethylglutaryl coenzyme A reductase inhibitors (stains), play a role in reducing ischemic events and mortality after AMI in general. In addition, pharmacological strategies to prevent adverse ventricular remodeling, such as ACE inhibitors and beta blockers, have proven beneficial in patients with post-AMI LVSD in particular. Due to these interventions, there has been a gradual decline in hospital mortality rates among this patient group. However, long-term mortality did not change over the two decades between 1975 and 1995 in one large, community-wide study [7].

* Corresponding author.
E-mail address: m-gheorghiade@northwestern.edu
(M. Gheorghiade).

The high mortality rates despite optimal reperfusion and medical therapy observed in patients with post-AMI LVSD may be related to an increased risk for postdischarge SCD. Although there is evidence that ACE inhibitors, beta blockers, and perhaps statins reduce its incidence, SCD remains an important cause of death in patients with post-AMI LVSD. The placement of a prophylactic implantable cardioverter defibrillator (ICD), a proven therapy for primary prevention of SCD in select populations, has not shown benefit if placed too soon after an AMI. Blockade of aldosterone receptors, however, has demonstrated efficacy in this particular patient population, especially in the immediate post-AMI period. This article discusses the epidemiology behind SCD in patients with post-AMI LVSD, the pathophysiology of aldosterone blockade in relation to SCD, the evidence behind aldosterone receptor blockade, safety concerns with the treatment, and, finally, a summary of available therapies for patients with post-AMI LVSD.

Sudden cardiac death

Much of what is known about the timing and risk of SCD after AMI in the presence of contemporary therapy comes from the Valsartan in Acute Myocardial Infarction Trial (VALIANT), published in 2003. This trial randomized 14,703 patients with AMI complicated by clinical or radiological HF, LVSD (LVEF $\leq$35% by echocardiography, contrast angiography, or $\leq$40% by radionuclide ventriculography), or both, to treatment with valsartan, captopril, or both within 0.5 to 10 days of AMI. Patients were required to have a systolic blood pressure >100 mm Hg and a serum creatinine (Cr) <2.5 mg/dL. There was 15% use of primary percutaneous coronary intervention (PCI) and 35% use of thrombolytic therapy. Adjunctive medical therapy for AMI included 91% aspirin, 70% beta blockers, but only 34% statins and 9% potassium-sparing diuretics. Mortality at 24 months was 20% and did not differ between groups compared [8]. In a subsequent analysis, the cause of death was reviewed by a central adjudication committee. SCD was defined as death that occurred "suddenly and unexpectedly" in a patient in otherwise stable condition who had not had premonitory HF, AMI, or other clear cause of death. SCD was combined with cardiac arrest with resuscitation to define the event rate in this analysis. A total of 7% of patients in this trial had such an event,

19% of whom had the event in the first 30 days post-AMI. The event rate was 1.4% per month during the first 30 days, and dropped to 0.5% per month during months 1 through 6, and to 0.14% 2 years post-AMI. During the critical first 30 days post-AMI, each reduction in LVEF by 5% was associated with a 21% increase in event rate. VALIANT established that the first 30 days post-AMI is a vulnerable period with the highest SCD and cardiac arrest-with-resuscitation rates, and that low LVEF can increase this risk dramatically [9].

In an attempt to reduce SCD during this vulnerable post-AMI period, the Defibrillator in Acute Myocardial Infarction Trial (DINAMIT) was published in 2004 [10]. In this trial, 674 post-AMI patients with LVEF $\leq$35% (assessed by angiography, radionuclide scanning, or echocardiography) and depressed heart-rate variability or elevated heart rate on 24-hour Holter monitoring were randomized to either an ICD or no ICD 6 to 40 days post-AMI. DINAMIT's adjunctive medication use was more aggressive than that of VALIANT, with 92% on antiplatelet agents, 87% on beta blockers, 95% on ACE inhibitors, and 78% on statin. In addition, there were slightly more primary PCIs at 36%, with similar use of thrombolytic therapy at 37%. After a mean follow-up of 30 months, overall mortality was 18% with no significant difference between treatment groups. Prespecified cause-of-death analysis was ascertained by the investigators at each site and derived from witnesses, family members, death certificates, hospital records, and autopsy reports, but not from ICD telemetry. Although there was a significant reduction in death from arrhythmia (hazard ratio [HR] 0.42, 95% CI, 0.22–0.83, $P =$ .009), this was offset by an increase in death from nonarrhythmic causes (HR 1.75, 95% CI, 1.11–2.76, $P =$ .02), primarily driven by cardiac nonarrhythmic causes (HR 1.72, 95% CI, 0.99–2.99, $P =$ .05). There were no deaths related to device implantation; however, in-hospital, device-related complications such as lead dislodgment, pneumothorax, and inappropriate shocks were documented in 25 patients.

In contrast with the findings in DINAMIT, the Multicenter Automatic Defibrillator Implantation Trial II (MADIT II) evaluated prophylactic ICD therapy in patients with prior AMI and LVEF $\leq$30%, and demonstrated that the rate of death due to arrhythmia was markedly reduced and the rate of nonarrhythmic death was not increased at a mean follow-up of 20 months [11]. These patients differed from DINAMIT patients in that they had a lower LVEF, did not have assessment of autonomic dysfunction, and, most importantly, were randomized a mean of 6.5 years after their most recent AMI. It is unclear why patients in DINAMIT who were assigned to ICD therapy had an increase in nonarrhythmic mortality. The presence of impaired autonomic dysfunction distinguishes DINAMIT patients from other post-AMI LVSD populations and may be a marker of risk for advanced HF. ICD therapy in these patients may therefore convert SCD into eventual death from pump failure. Additionally, inappropriate shocks and placement of an ICD itself may lead to negative remodeling and worsened HF. Whatever the mechanism, placement of an ICD for primary prevention of SCD within the first 40 days of AMI is recommended against by the ACC/AHA guidelines for the management of patients with ST-segment-elevation MI and the ACC/AHA/ESC guidelines for the prevention of SCD [12,13]. With failure of proven therapies to prevent SCD in patients with post-AMI LVSD, there has been a need for newer therapies. Aldosterone receptor blockade has proved to be an effective experimental and clinical strategy in this patient group.

The role of aldosterone in myocardial infarction

Aldosterone is implicated not only in fluid and potassium balance, but also in post-AMI left ventricular (LV) remodeling. Depressed cardiac function after AMI leads to a series of neurohormonal reflexes that activate the sympathetic nervous system and the renin-angiotensin-aldosterone systems. These reflexes are initially adaptive to preserve mean arterial pressure, but prolonged neurohormonal activation eventually becomes maladaptive and leads to increased myocardial oxygen demand, progressive myocardial injury, ventricular dysfunction and ultimately HF [14,15]. Alterations in ventricular architecture result, involving infarcted and noninfarcted areas of the left ventricle, and these alterations lead to contractile dysfunction, fibrosis, progressive dilation, hypertrophy and distortion of the ventricular cavity, known as LV remodeling [16]. LV remodeling and neurohormonal activation are associated with increased risk for ventricular arrhythmias and SCD. Aldosterone has been found to be elevated in patients with LVSD and associated with poor outcomes in the chronic [17] and acute MI settings [18].

Aldosterone blockade, alone or in combination with ACE inhibitors, has been associated with many potentially favorable effects on post-AMI LV remodeling in a wide range of animal models. These include reduced collagen deposition, norepinephrine levels, interstitial fibrosis, hypertrophy, LV dimensions and increased LVEF [19–25]. Table 1 outlines the mechanisms of the deleterious effects of aldosterone in the AMI setting and the efficacy of aldosterone blockade in reversing these effects.

Endothelial dysfunction

In experimental models, aldosterone has been found to inhibit the production of nitrite oxide

Table 1
Potential deleterious mechanisms, anatomical effects, and possible clinical consequences of aldosterone on the cardiovascular system, beyond fluid and potassium balance

Mechanisms	Anatomical effects	Possible clinical consequences
↓ Endothelial-derived nitric oxide [26]	Vasoconstriction	Ischemia
↑ Oxidative stress [31]	Inflammation and fibrosis	LV remodeling, HF
Collagen deposition [32–34]	Fibrosis, stiffness, and distortion of the myocardial structure	LV remodeling, HF
Vascular inflammation [39]	Myocardial fibrosis and necrosis	LV remodeling, HF
Myocardial apoptosis [46]	Myocytes loss	LV remodeling, HF
↓ Baroreceptor sensitivity and Reflex function [40,41]	↑ Heart rate variability, arrhythmias	SCD
↓ Myocardial uptake of norepinephrine [42]	Arrhythmias	SCD
↑ Action potential duration [44]	Arrhythmias	SCD
↓ Fibrinolysis [45]	Thrombophilic state	Ischemia, necrosis
↑ Platelet activation [45]	Thrombophilic state	Ischemia, necrosis

Abbreviations: LV, left ventricular; ↑, increased; ↓, decreased.

(NO) in peripheral vessels [26,27]. This reduction in NO causes vasoconstriction and increased vascular tone that, in turn, leads to reduced myocardial perfusion and, eventually, myocardial injury [28,29]. The nonselective aldosterone blocker spironolactone seems to improve endothelial dysfunction and normalize these deleterious effects in animal and human studies [30].

Aldosterone, in combination with a high-salt environment, seems to promote oxidative stress by increasing the activity of reduced-form nicotinamide adenine dinucleotide phosphate oxidase. This increase leads to the production of superoxide radicals, endothelial damage and vasoconstriction, and, eventually, inflammation and fibrosis in animal models—effects that are attenuated by spironolactone [31].

Collagen synthesis

There is increasing evidence that aldosterone may exert adverse affects on the vascular and myocardial matrix by increasing collagen synthesis. Although collagen has important structural properties, its overproduction (particularly types I and III) is associated with stiffness and distortion of the tissue structure [32–34]. This mechanism explains, at least in part, the role of aldosterone in LV remodeling post-AMI [35–37]. Still, after 8 weeks of spironolactone treatment in patients with chronic HF, reversal of collagen synthesis was demonstrated by a 20% reduction of pro-collagen type III N-terminal amino peptide (PIIINP, a biomarker of vascular collagen turnover) [38].

Inflammation

Vascular inflammation is another potential effect of aldosterone-induced myocardial injury and fibrosis. There is evidence that aldosterone infusion in salt-loaded rats induced severe coronary inflammatory lesions, resulting in fibrosis, focal ischemia, and necrosis [39]. These structural alterations may also be responsible for the decreased arterial compliance in patients with hypertension [32]. These phenomena can be altered after 8 weeks of treatment with eplerenone, a selective aldosterone receptor blocker [39].

Autonomic nervous system

Aldosterone has been shown in animal [40] and human [41] models to decrease baroreceptor sensitivity and reflex function. Furthermore, aldosterone has been shown to block myocardial uptake of norepinephrine in rats by 24%, which

may reduce heart-rate variability and, potentially, catecholamine-induced arrhythmias [42]. These findings are consistent with data from patients with chronic, stable HF in whom spironolactone, in addition to standard medical therapy, increased myocardial norepinephrine uptake, reduced ventricular arrhythmias on 24-hour ambulatory electrocardiography, and improved heart-rate variability compared with similar patients given placebo [38,43]. Although its potential pro-arrhythmic effects are not completely understood, growing literature shows that aldosterone may influence electrical properties of cardiac myocytes by increasing action potential duration by altering calcium channel current density [44].

Other mechanisms

Other potentially deleterious effects of aldosterone have been shown in human and animal models, including inhibition of fibrinolysis and platelet activation, which promotes the hypercoagulable state observed in the post-AMI setting [45], and myocardial apoptosis as an adjunctive mechanism of LV remodeling [46]. Once again, aldosterone receptor blockade attenuated these processes [47].

Experimental evidence in humans

Modena and colleagues [48] studied the effects of aldosterone suppression with potassium canrenoate (50 mg/d) on collagen synthesis and LV dimensions. This small, randomized, placebo-controlled study enrolled 46 patients after recent thrombolysis for anterior AMI who were also given ACE inhibitors at the time of discharge. Serum PIIINP, a marker of collagen synthesis, and LV diameter were significantly lower in the canrenoate group compared with placebo at 3, 6, and 12 months.

The reduction in collagen synthesis and attenuation of remodeling may slow progression of diastolic dysfunction after AMI. Echocardiographic studies demonstrated that in AMI patients not receiving, or unsuitable for, reperfusion therapy, canreoate (25 mg/d) in addition to captopril resulted in lower LV end-systolic volumes (LVESV), higher LVEF, higher E-wave-to-A-wave (E/A) ratios, and lower isovolumetric relaxation (IVRT) times compared with placebo after 6 months in a larger randomized pilot study [49].

In a study by Hayashi and colleagues [50], 134 patients with anterior AMI were assigned to enalapril and spironolactone (25 mg/d) versus enalapril alone immediately after revascularization. At 30 days, the combination therapy arm had a significantly greater increase in LVEF (+7.2% versus +4.46%, P < .05), and decreases in LV end-diastolic (LVEDVI) and end-systolic (LVESDI) volume indices, transcardiac extraction of aldosterone, and PIIINP levels compared with the enalapril-only group, suggesting a greater protective effect of combination therapy against post-AMI LV remodeling. These small clinical trials with promising results for the improvement of LV remodeling and reduction in electrical instability, summarized in Table 2 led to a large, randomized, controlled trial evaluating hard endpoints for aldosterone receptor blockade in high-risk, post-AMI LVSD patients.

Aldosterone blockade with eplerenone

The Eplerenone Post-Acute Myocardial Infarction Heart Failure Efficacy and Survival Study (EPHESUS) trial, published in 2003, was a multicenter, double-blind, placebo-controlled, international trial of 6,632 patients with AMI complicated by LVSD (LVEF ≤40% by echocardiography, radionuclide angiography, or contrast angiography), with symptoms of HF (pulmonary rales, pulmonary edema, or presence of a third heart sound) or diabetes who were randomized to eplerenone, a selective aldosterone receptor blocker, or placebo within 3 to 14 days of AMI [51]. Eplerenone was started at 25 mg/d and increased to a maximum of 50 mg/d after 4 weeks. In patients with diabetes and post-AMI LVSD, symptoms of HF were not required, because outcomes in such patients compared with those in nondiabetic patients with post-AMI LVSD with symptoms of HF were similar [52]. Patients with a serum Cr >2.5 mg/dL and those with evidence of serum potassium >5.0 mEq/L were excluded. Standard therapy included reperfusion (45%), ACE inhibitors or ARBs (86%), beta blockers (75%), aspirin (88%), statins (47%), and diuretics (60%). After a mean follow-up of 16 months, eplerenone significantly reduced the risk of all-cause mortality by 15% (14% versus 17%, P = .008) and cardiovascular (CV) mortality/CV hospitalization by 13% (27% versus 30%, P = .002), both primary end points in the study. Death from CV causes was reduced by 17% (12% versus 15%, P = .005), driven by a 21% reduction in SCD (4.8% versus 6.1%, P = .03). There was a nonsignificant reduction in hospitalization for CV events of 9% (18% versus 20%, P = .09),

driven by a 15% reduction in HF admissions (10% versus 12%, P = .03) (Fig. 1).

The critical period of 30 days after AMI, when the risk of SCD is greatest, was studied in a prespecified analysis of EPHESUS [53]. Analysis of primary endpoints demonstrated that, compared with placebo, eplerenone reduced all-cause mortality by 31% (3.2% versus 4.6%, P = .004), and nonsignificantly reduced death from CV causes/CV hospitalization. Using Kaplan-Meyer analysis, a significant treatment effect was seen starting at 10 days into treatment. Death from CV causes was reduced by 32% (3.0% versus 4.4%, P = .003), again driven by a 37% reduction in SCD (0.9% versus 1.4%, P = .03) (Fig. 2). This 1.4% risk of SCD within 30 days post-AMI in the placebo arm is the same as that in the treatment arms of VALIANT, making the reduction to 0.9% by eplerenone of significant clinical relevance.

In the post-AMI patients with LVEF ≤30%, further reductions in the primary and secondary endpoints were observed with eplerenone in a post hoc analysis of EPHESUS [54]. Of the 6,632 patients in EPHESUS, 2,106 (32%) had an LVEF of ≤30%, and similar baseline characteristics between treatment groups, but more diabetes, HF, and prior AMI history than the overall EPHESUS population. Compared with the overall placebo-treated EPHESUS population, placebo-treated patients with LVEF ≤30% had a higher incidence of all-cause death (24.0% versus 16.7%), CV mortality/CV hospitalization (40.9% versus 30.0%), and SCD (9.7% versus 6.1%). In this high-risk group, compared with placebo, eplerenone administration was associated with a 21% reduction in all-cause mortality (20% versus 24%, P = .12) and a 21% reduction of CV mortality/CV hospitalization (34% versus 41%, P = .001). At the conclusion of the study, CV mortality was reduced by 23% (17% versus 21%, P = .008) and SCD was reduced by 33% (6.8% versus 9.7%, P = .01). Nonfatal hospitalization for HF was reduced by 20% (15% versus 17%, P = .75) but death due to progressive HF was reduced nonsignificantly (4.7% versus 5.6%, P = .28) (Fig. 3). Compared to the overall EPHESUS population, the patients with LVEF ≤30% had a higher event rate but derived the greatest benefit with eplerenone (Fig. 4).

EPHESUS established the mortality benefit of aldosterone receptor blockade with eplerenone in patients with post-AMI LVSD and either symptoms of HF or the presence of diabetes. The CV

Table 2
Overview of clinical trials on aldosterone blockade in patients with left ventricular systolic dysfunction after an acute myocardial infarction

Study	Inclusion criteria	Number of patients studied	Randomized groups	Follow-up	Primary end point(s)	Main finding
Modena et al [48]	Anterior AMI, r-tPA within 6 hours of chest pain, ACE I after randomization	46	Potassium canrenoate (50 mg/d) versus placebo on discharge following AMI	Months 3, 6, 12	Measurement of PIIINP and LV volume	Significant reduction in PIIINP in canrenoate-treated group at 3, 6, and 12 months, significant reduction in LV volume in canrenoate-treated group at 6 and 12 months
Di Pasquale et al [49]	Anterior AMI, without reperfusion	187	Potassium canrenoate (25 mg/d) plus captopril versus placebo plus captopril immediately following AMI	Days 10, 90, 180	Measurement of LVESV, LVEF, LVEDD, E/A ratio, E decal time, IVRT	Improvement in LVESV, LVEF, E/A ratio, and IVRT
Hayashi et al [50]	Anterior AMI, successful reperfusion within 24 hours	134	Spironolactone (25 mg/d) plus enalapril versus placebo plus enalapril immediately after revascularization for AMI	1 month	Measurement of PIIINP, LVEF, LVEDVI, LVESVI	Transcardiac aldosterone extraction reduced, PIIINP levels suppressed in treatment group, LVEF increase greater, LVEDVI increase suppressed, LVESVI decrease greater in treatment groups compared with placebo
EPHESUS [51]	AMI, LVEF ≤40% and either HF symptoms or DM	6,632	Eplerenone (25-50 mg/d) versus placebo plus optimal medical therapy 3-14 days following AMI	16 months	Time to death from any cause and time to death from any CV cause or hospitalization for CV event	15% all-cause mortality risk reduction ($P = .008$), 13% CV mortality or CV hospitalization risk reduction ($P = .002$)

Abbreviations: ACE I, angiotensin-converting enzyme inhibitor; DM, diabetes mellitus; EPHESUS, Eplerenone Post-Acute Myocardial Infarction Heart Failure Efficacy and Survival Study; IVRT, isovolemic relaxation time; LVEDD, left ventricular end diastolic dimension; LVEDVI, left ventricular end diastolic volume index; LVESV, left ventricular end systolic volume; LVESVI, left ventricular end systolic volume index; r-tPA, recombinant tissue plasminogen activator.

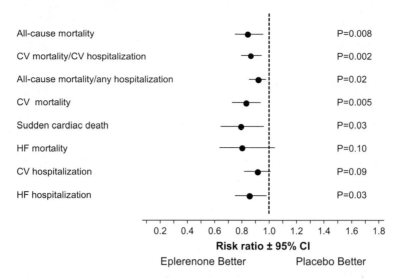

Fig. 1. Relative risks of primary and secondary end points in EPHESUS. (*Adapted from* Pitt B, Remme W, Zannad F, et al. Eplerenone, a selective aldosterone blocker, in patients with left ventricular dysfunction after myocardial infarction. N Engl J Med 2003;348:1309–21.)

mortality reduction is predominantly driven by reductions in SCD, and this SCD reduction is seen as early as 10 days after therapy. The benefit of eplerenone is greatest in those patients with the worst LVSD. EPHESUS patients were on standard medical therapy, with ACE inhibitors or ARBs (85%), beta blockers (75%), and statins (47%). In addition, 45% of patients had reperfusion therapy to limit the infarct size, and 89% were receiving antiplatelet therapy with aspirin. Accordingly, eplerenone was effective in patients who were already receiving evidence-based therapy for CAD and LVSD, including ACE inhibitors and beta blockers.

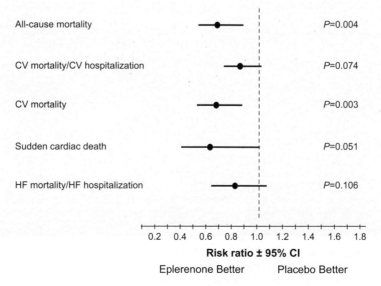

Fig. 2. Relative risks of mortality and morbidity at 30 days in all EPHESUS patients. (*Adapted from* Pitt B, White H, Nicolau J, et al. Eplerenone reduces mortality 30 days after randomization following acute myocardial infarction in patients with left ventricular systolic dysfunction and heart failure. J Am Coll Cardiol 2005;46:425–31.)

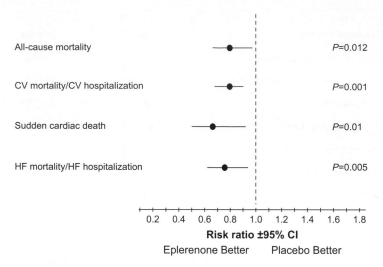

Fig. 3. Relative risks of mortality and morbidity in EPHESUS patients with left ventricular ejection fraction of 30% or less. (*Adapted from* Pitt B, Gheorghiade M, Zannad F, et al. Evaluation of eplerenone in the subgroup of EPHESUS patients with baseline left ventricular ejection fraction < or = 30%. Eur J Heart Fail 2006;8:295–301.)

Safety concerns with eplerenone

Hemodynamics

At the time EPHESUS was planned, there was little experience with the use of aldosterone receptor blockade during the early hours after AMI and hypotension seemed to be one of the major concerns, given the high-risk post-AMI population. Thus, it was decided to delay the administration of eplerenone until patients were hemodynamically stable between 3 to 14 days after myocardial infarction. At 30 days after randomization, placebo-treated patients experienced significantly greater systolic and diastolic blood

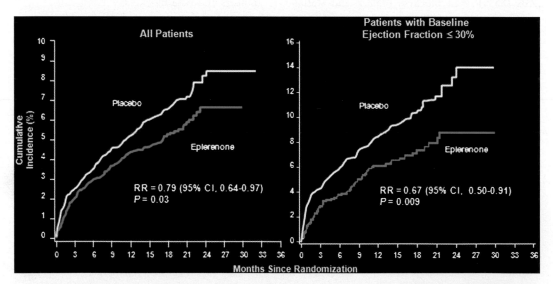

Fig. 4. Relative risk (RR) of sudden cardiac death in the eplerenone and in the placebo group in the main EPHESUS trial compared with the subgroup analysis of patients with left ventricular ejection fraction ≤30%. (*Adapted from* Pitt B, Remme W, Zannad F, et al. Eplerenone, a selective aldosterone blocker, in patients with left ventricular dysfunction after myocardial infarction. N Engl J Med 2003;348:1309–21 and Pitt B, Gheorghiade M, Zannad F, et al. Evaluation of eplerenone in the subgroup of EPHESUS patients with baseline left ventricular ejection fraction < or = 30%. Eur J Heart Fail 2006;8:295–301.)

pressure elevation than patients treated with eplerenone (4.0/2.9 versus 2.4/1.7 mm Hg, $P<.01$), a magnitude that may not be clinically significant. This effect was sustained at 1 year (8/4 versus 5/3 mm Hg, $P<.01$). No significant change in body weight was observed at 1 year. These data, summarized in Fig. 5, suggest that the antihypertensive effect of eplerenone is minimal even with background therapy of ACE inhibitors and beta blockers and may be used early post-AMI. Now that it is known that administration within 3 to 14 days of AMI does not adversely lower blood pressure, it is unclear if earlier administration of eplerenone will give greater benefit, by preventing SCD and worsening pump failure. Although Hayashi and colleagues [50] demonstrated benefits in LV function and remodeling with aldosterone receptor blockade as early as 1 hour after revascularization, the translation to clinical endpoints requires prospective evaluation in larger trials.

Renal function

In EPHESUS, serum Cr increased by 0.02 mg/dL in the placebo group and 0.06 mg/dL in the eplerenone group ($P<.001$) at 1 year. EPHESUS excluded patients with serum Cr >2.5 mg/dL. With a mean age of enrollment of 64, a serum Cr > 2.5 mg/dL translates to an estimated glomerular filtration rate (eGFR) of ≤ 29 mL/min/1.73 m^2 for men and ≤ 22 mL/min/1.73 m^2 for women, using the modification of diet in renal

disease (MDRD) formula. Calculation and close monitoring of the eGFR rather than serum Cr may be a more reliable way of predicting CV outcome, especially in the elderly and in women: eGFR is significantly worse with age and female gender for any given Cr level [55]. In fact, analysis of VALIANT demonstrated that, for eGFR <81 mL/min/1.73 m^2, there was a hazard ratio for death or nonfatal CV outcomes of 1.1 for every 10-unit reduction in eGFR, independent of treatment assignment [56]. Eplerenone should be discontinued when the eGFR approaches 30 mL/min/1.73 m^2, and use of other nephrotoxins such as nonsteroidal anti-inflammatory drugs should be avoided.

Hyperkalemia

The incidence of serious hyperkalemia (serum potassium ≥ 6.0 mEq/dL) in EPHESUS was greater in patients treated with eplerenone than with placebo (5.5 versus 3.9%, $P = .002$) at 1 year. Among patients with a baseline eGFR <50 mL/min, calculated using the Cockcroft-Gault formula, incidence of serious hyperkalemia was 10.1% in the eplerenone group and 5.9% in the placebo group ($P = .006$). Corresponding rates for eGFR ≥ 50 mL/min were 4.6% and 3.5%, respectively ($P = .04$). Within the first 30 days of treatment, serum potassium increased by 0.24 mmol/L in the eplerenone group and 0.17 mmol/L in the placebo group ($P<.001$). However, in this trial after adjudication, no deaths were attributed

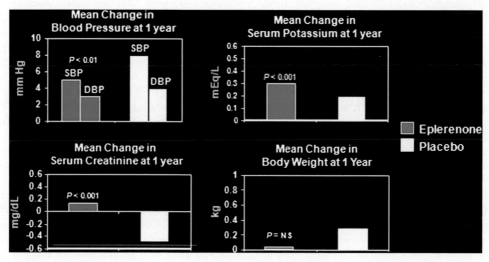

Fig. 5. Effects of eplerenone on blood pressure, serum potassium, serum Cr, and body weight in EPHESUS patients at 1 year. (*Adapted from* Pitt B, Remme W, Zannad F, et al. Eplerenone, a selective aldosterone blocker, in patients with left ventricular dysfunction after myocardial infarction. N Engl J Med 2003;348:1309–21.)

to hyperkalemia. Hypokalemia (serum potassium ≤3.5 mEq/L) may be as great if not a greater risk than hyperkalemia in patients with HF [57] and occurred less frequently in eplerenone-treated patients than in placebo-treated patients (8.4% versus 13.1%, $P < .001$).

In real-world practice, care must be taken with aldosterone receptor blockade in patients with post-AMI LVSD. The Randomized Aldactone Evaluation Study (RALES) trial was a pivotal study published in 1999 that showed a mortality benefit of spironalactone in patients with an LVEF ≤35%, with severe (NYHA Class III-IV), chronic HF being treated with ACE inhibitors, if tolerated, and a loop diuretic [58]. Publication of this trial led to a more widespread use of aldosterone receptor blockade in patients with LVSD. A population-based, time-series analysis was performed using health care databases and hospitalization records obtained from the Canadian Institute of Health Information Discharge Abstract Database and the Ontario Drug Benefits Program of all patients 65 years of age or older in Ontario, Canada. The accuracy of the hospitalization records had not been previously established for hyperkalemia. This study analyzed the rates of spironolactone use and hyperkalemia in patients with HF treated with ACE inhibitors before and after publication of RALES [59]. There was an increase in prescription of spironolactone by a factor of about 5 from 1999 compared with late 2001. The rate of hospital admissions involving a diagnosis of hyperkalemia increased from 4.0/1000 patients to 11.0/1000 patients from 1999 to late 2001. During the same period, the mortality in patients admitted with hyperkalemia increased from 0.7/1000 patients to 2.0/1000 patients.

Since the authors had no knowledge of the serum potassium during hospitalization and did not adjust for comorbidities, it is far from clear whether this substantial increase in mortality was related to hyperkalemia caused by spironolactone use. In fact, hyperkalemia has been reported as a major marker for severity of HF, independent of spironolactone use [60]. RALES excluded patients with a serum Cr of >2.5 mg/dL or a serum potassium of >5.0 mEq/L. RALES followed laboratory measurements, including serum potassium every 4 weeks for the first 12 weeks, then every 3 months for up to 1 year, and every 6 months thereafter. EPHESUS had the same serum Cr and potassium exclusion criteria, and monitored potassium and Cr levels 48 hours after initiation,

at 1, 4, and 5 weeks, at all scheduled study visits, and within 1 week after any change in dose. Accordingly, when simple monitoring criteria are followed, the rate of hyperkalemia in patients already receiving ACE inhibitors and beta blockers, as was the case in EPHESUS, is low. The rates of serious hyperkalemia in the treatment arms compared with placebo in RALES and EPHESUS were 2% versus 1%, and 5.5% versus 3.9%, respectively.

Recommendations for prevention of SCD in patients with post-AMI LVSD

Patients with post-AMI LVSD present at a critical juncture between acute coronary event and HF. The failure to recognize this syndrome as a distinct entity that needs therapeutic interventions tailored accordingly may, at least in part, explain the questionable results of the recent DINAMIT trial that, as previously discussed, failed to demonstrate any benefit with early ICD implantation in patients with post-AMI LVSD. The available data and ACC/AHA guidelines suggest that several treatment strategies should be implemented in an effort to improve outcomes in this patient population. These treatment strategies are briefly discussed below. The guidelines for ST-segment-elevation MI (STEMI) [12], unstable angina, non-ST-segment-elevation MI (UA/NSTEMI) [61], and prevention of SCD [13] are cited and summarized in Table 3.

With LVSD being such a poor prognostic factor in post-AMI patients, assessment of LVEF is critical in all patients with AMI. This can be done using many modalities, including contrast angiography if coronary angiography is performed, radionuclide angiography, or echocardiography. The ACC/AHA guidelines for the management of STEMI give LVEF assessment a class I indication for all post-AMI patients. A similar recommendation is given in the guidelines for the management of UA/NSTEMI.

Aldosterone receptor blockade is beneficial in patients with post-MI LVSD who are receiving other therapies such as reperfusion therapy, antiplatelet therapy, beta blockers [62,63], ACE inhibitors [64–66], and ARBs [8,67]. The importance of adrenergic blockade, including beta blockers, ACE inhibitors, and ARBs, in this setting is reviewed elsewhere in this issue of the *Cardiology Clinics.*

There is increasing evidence that statins, through the improvement they effect in endothelial

Table 3
Class I indications for assessment and treatment of myocardial infarction and concomitant left ventricular dysfunction (adapted from [12,13,60])

Intervention	Class I indication
LVEF assessment	
STEMI	LVEF should be measured in all STEMI patients (*Level of Evidence: B*)
UA/NSTEMI	A noninvasive test (echocardiogram or radionuclide angiogram) is recommended to evaluate LV function in patients with definite ACS who are not scheduled for coronary angiography and left ventriculography (*Level of Evidence: B*)
Beta blockers	
STEMI	Patients with moderate or severe LV failure should receive beta-blocker therapy with a gradual titration scheme (*Level of Evidence: B*)
UA/NSTEMI	Patients recovering from UA/NSTEMI with moderate or severe LV failure should receive beta-blocker therapy with a gradual titration scheme (*Level of Evidence: B*)
ACE inhibitors	
STEMI	An ACE inhibitor should be prescribed at discharge for all patients without contraindications after STEMI (*Level of Evidence: A*)
UA/NSTEMI	ACE inhibitors should be given and continued indefinitely for patients recovering from UA/NSTEMI with HF, LV dysfunction (LVEF <0.40), hypertension, or diabetes mellitus, unless contraindicated (*Level of Evidence: A*)
ARBs	
STEMI	An ARB should be administered or prescribed at discharge to STEMI patients who are intolerant of an ACE inhibitor and have either clinical or radiological signs of HF and LVEF <0.40. Valsartan and candesartan have established efficacy for this recommendation (*Level of Evidence: B*)
UA/NSTEMI	An ARB should be administered or prescribed at discharge to UA/NSTEMI patients who are intolerant to ACE inhibitors and have either clinical or radiological signs of HF and LVEF <0.40 (*Level of Evidence: A*)
Aldosterone receptor blockers	
STEMI	Long-term aldosterone blockade should be prescribed for post-STEMI patients without significant renal dysfunction (Cr should be ≤2.5 mg/dL in men and <2.0 mg/dL in women) or hyperkalemia (potassium should be ≤5.0 mEq/L) who are already receiving therapeutic doses of an ACE inhibitor, have an LVEF of ≤0.40, and have either symptomatic HF or diabetes (*Level of Evidence: A*)
UA/NSTEMI	Long-term aldosterone receptor blockade should be prescribed for UA/NSTEMI patients without significant renal dysfunction (estimated Cr clearance should be > 30 mL/min) or hyperkalemia (potassium should be ≤5 mEq/L) who are already receiving therapeutic doses of an ACE inhibitor, have an LVEF ≤0.40, and have either symptomatic HF or diabetes mellitus (*Level of Evidence: A*)
ICDs	ICD therapy is recommended for primary prevention to reduce total mortality by a reduction in SCD in patients with LV dysfunction because of prior MI who are at least 40 days post-MI, have an LVEF ≤30%–40%, are NYHA-functional class II or III receiving chronic optimal medical therapy, and who have reasonable expectation of survival with a good functional status for more than 1 year (*Level of Evidence: A*)

function, plaque stabilization, and lipid profile, may contribute to the reduction in SCD in patients with CAD [68,69]. Although most of the data are retrospective in nature, it appears that, irrespective of their exact mechanism of action, statins have shown a significant reduction in ventricular arrhythmias [70–73]. Although no specific ACC/AHA recommendation exists regarding statins in post-AMI LVSD, statins are recommended in all post-MI patients irrespective of their LV function.

Table 3 summarizes the ACC/AHA recommendations for care of patients with post-AMI LVSD.

ICD implantation, although found to improve mortality long-term, does not seem to be beneficial in the early phase post-AMI, as suggested by the MADIT-II and DINAMIT trials. Accordingly, the ACC/AHA/ESC gives a class I recommendation for the prophylactic implantation of an ICD in these patients, but only beyond 40 days post-AMI [13].

The ACC/AHA guidelines for the management of STEMI and UA/NSTEMI give aldosterone receptor blockers, such as eplerenone, a class I indication for hospital management and secondary prevention in patients with post-AMI LVSD. Despite this recommendation, the use of aldosterone receptor blockade is sparse in post-AMI LVSD in clinical practice. Recent analysis of the 48,612 patients in the Organized Program to Initiate Life-Saving Treatment in Hospitalized Patients with Heart Failure (OPTIMIZE-HF) registry of patients hospitalized for acute heart failure demonstrated that, in patients with LVSD, defined as LVEF ≤40% and CAD with prior revascularization procedures, only 11% were taking an aldosterone receptor blocker of some kind, while 65% were taking a beta blocker, 59% an ACE inhibitor or ARB, and 49% a statin (unpublished data). Efforts need to be placed to initiate this life-saving medication during the critical period after AMI and before discharge.

Summary

AMI is commonly associated with LVSD and HF, and confers substantial mortality and morbidity. Several adjunctive therapies have proved to reduce mortality and morbidity, including antiplatelet agents, statins, beta blockers, ACE inhibitors, ARBs for patients intolerant of ACE inhibitors, and ICD implantation at least 40 days after AMI. Aldosterone has many deleterious effects and is elevated in patients with post-AMI LVSD. Eplerenone, by blocking the aldosterone receptor, is a new therapy for these high-risk patients that has proved to reduce mortality and morbidity when used in conjunction with beta-blocker and ACE-inhibitor therapy. Eplerenone reduces SCD in the early post-AMI period (<30 days), particularly in patients with a LVEF ≤30%. These patients with severe LVSD are at very high risk of SCD despite receiving beta-blocker and ACE-inhibitor/ARB therapy.

Although ICD therapy is known to reduce the rate of SCD in patients with HF and post-AMI LVSD, it does not seem to be effective within the first 40 days post-AMI. Aldosterone receptor-blocking agents are beneficial with proper patient selection (serum Cr <2.5 mg/dL, potassium <5.0 mEq/L) and close monitoring of renal function and serum potassium concentration, particularly in patients who are receiving ACE inhibitors or ARBs and have diabetes.

References

[1] Rosamond W, Flegal K, Friday G, et al. Heart disease and stroke statistics—2007 update: a report from the American Heart Association Statistics Committee and Stroke Statistics Subcommittee. Circulation 2007;115:e69–171.

[2] Hasdai D, Topol EJ, Kilaru R, et al. Frequency, patient characteristics, and outcomes of mild-to-moderate heart failure complicating ST-segment elevation acute myocardial infarction: lessons from 4 international fibrinolytic therapy trials. Am Heart J 2003;145:73–9.

[3] Steg PG, Dabbous OH, Feldman LJ, et al. Determinants and prognostic impact of heart failure complicating acute coronary syndromes: observations from the Global Registry of Acute Coronary Events (GRACE). Circulation 2004;109:494–9.

[4] Wu AH, Parsons L, Every NR, et al. Hospital outcomes in patients presenting with congestive heart failure complicating acute myocardial infarction: a report from the Second National Registry of Myocardial Infarction (NRMI-2). J Am Coll Cardiol 2002;40:1389–94.

[5] Velazquez EJ, Francis GS, Armstrong PW, et al. An international perspective on heart failure and left ventricular systolic dysfunction complicating myocardial infarction: the VALIANT registry. Eur Heart J 2004;25:1911–9.

[6] Spencer FA, Meyer TE, Gore JM, et al. Heterogeneity in the management and outcomes of patients with acute myocardial infarction complicated by heart failure: the National Registry of Myocardial Infarction. Circulation 2002;105:2605–10.

[7] Spencer FA, Meyer TE, Goldberg RJ, et al. Twenty year trends (1975–1995) in the incidence, in-hospital and long-term death rates associated with heart failure complicating acute myocardial infarction: a community-wide perspective. J Am Coll Cardiol 1999; 34:1378–87.

[8] Pfeffer MA, McMurray JJ, Velazquez EJ, et al. Valsartan, captopril, or both in myocardial infarction complicated by heart failure, left ventricular dysfunction, or both. N Engl J Med 2003;349: 1893–906.

[9] Solomon SD, Zelenkofske S, McMurray JJ, et al. Sudden death in patients with myocardial infarction and left ventricular dysfunction, heart failure, or both. N Engl J Med 2005;352:2581–8.

[10] Hohnloser SH, Kuck KH, Dorian P, et al. Prophylactic use of an implantable cardioverter-defibrillator after acute myocardial infarction. N Engl J Med 2004;351:2481–8.

[11] Moss AJ, Zareba W, Hall WJ, et al. Prophylactic implantation of a defibrillator in patients with myocardial infarction and reduced ejection fraction. N Engl J Med 2002;346:877–83.

[12] Antman EM, Anbe DT, Armstrong PW, et al. ACC/AHA guidelines for the management of patients with ST-elevation myocardial infarction–executive summary: a report of the American College of Cardiology/American Heart Association Task Force on Practice Guidelines (Writing Committee to Revise the 1999 Guidelines for the Management of Patients With Acute Myocardial Infarction). Circulation 2004;110:588–636.

[13] Zipes DP, Camm AJ, Borggrefe M, et al. ACC/AHA/ESC 2006 guidelines for management of patients with ventricular arrhythmias and the prevention of sudden cardiac death: a report of the American College of Cardiology/American Heart Association Task Force and the European Society of Cardiology Committee for Practice Guidelines (Writing Committee to Develop Guidelines for Management of Patients With Ventricular Arrhythmias and the Prevention of Sudden Cardiac Death). J Am Coll Cardiol 2006;48:e247–346.

[14] Udelson JE, Patten RD, Konstam MA. New concepts in post-infarction ventricular remodeling. Rev Cardiovasc Med 2003;4(Suppl 3):S3–12.

[15] Harrison TR, Kasper DL. Harrison's principles of internal medicine. 16th edn. New York: McGraw-Hill Medical Pub. Division; 2005.

[16] Pfeffer MA, Braunwald E. Ventricular remodeling after myocardial infarction. Experimental observations and clinical implications. Circulation 1990;81: 1161–72.

[17] Swedberg K, Eneroth P, Kjekshus J, et al. Hormones regulating cardiovascular function in patients with severe congestive heart failure and their relation to mortality. CONSENSUS Trial Study Group. Circulation 1990;82:1730–6.

[18] Beygui F, Collet JP, Benoliel JJ, et al. High plasma aldosterone levels on admission are associated with death in patients presenting with acute ST-elevation myocardial infarction. Circulation 2006;114: 2604–10.

[19] Delyani JA, Robinson EL, Rudolph AE. Effect of a selective aldosterone receptor antagonist in myocardial infarction. Am J Physiol Heart Circ Physiol 2001;281:H647–54.

[20] Suzuki G, Morita H, Mishima T, et al. Effects of long-term monotherapy with eplerenone, a novel aldosterone blocker, on progression of left ventricular dysfunction and remodeling in dogs with heart failure. Circulation 2002;106:2967–72.

[21] Fraccarollo D, Galuppo P, Hildemann S, et al. Additive improvement of left ventricular remodeling and neurohormonal activation by aldosterone receptor blockade with eplerenone and ACE inhibition in rats with myocardial infarction. J Am Coll Cardiol 2003;42:1666–73.

[22] Wang D, Liu YH, Yang XP, et al. Role of a selective aldosterone blocker in mice with chronic heart failure. J Card Fail 2004;10:67–73.

[23] Masson S, Staszewsky L, Annoni G, et al. Eplerenone, a selective aldosterone blocker, improves diastolic function in aged rats with small-to-moderate myocardial infarction. J Card Fail 2004;10: 433–41.

[24] Silvestre JS, Heymes C, Oubenaissa A, et al. Activation of cardiac aldosterone production in rat myocardial infarction: effect of angiotensin II receptor blockade and role in cardiac fibrosis. Circulation 1999;99:2694–701.

[25] Perrier E, Kerfant BG, Lalevee N, et al. Mineralocorticoid receptor antagonism prevents the electrical remodeling that precedes cellular hypertrophy after myocardial infarction. Circulation 2004;110:776–83.

[26] Ikeda U, Kanbe T, Nakayama I, et al. Aldosterone inhibits nitric oxide synthesis in rat vascular smooth muscle cells induced by interleukin-1 beta. Eur J Pharmacol 1995;290:69–73.

[27] Fleming I, Busse R. NO: the primary EDRF. J Mol Cell Cardiol 1999;31:5–14.

[28] Wang J, Seyedi N, Xu XB, et al. Defective endothelium-mediated control of coronary circulation in conscious dogs after heart failure. Am J Physiol 1994;266:H670–80.

[29] Qi XL, Stewart DJ, Gosselin H, et al. Improvement of endocardial and vascular endothelial function on myocardial performance by captopril treatment in postinfarct rat hearts. Circulation 1999;100: 1338–45.

[30] Bauersachs J, Heck M, Fraccarollo D, et al. Addition of spironolactone to angiotensin-converting enzyme inhibition in heart failure improves endothelial vasomotor dysfunction: role of vascular superoxide anion formation and endothelial nitric oxide synthase expression. J Am Coll Cardiol 2002;39:351–8.

[31] Sun Y, Zhang J, Lu L, et al. Aldosterone-induced inflammation in the rat heart: role of oxidative stress. Am J Pathol 2002;161:1773–81.

[32] Duprez D, De Buyzere M, Rietzschel ER, et al. Aldosterone and vascular damage. Curr Hypertens Rep 2000;2:327–34.

[33] Sutton MG, Sharpe N. Left ventricular remodeling after myocardial infarction: pathophysiology and therapy. Circulation 2000;101:2981–8.

[34] Brilla CG, Zhou G, Matsubara L, et al. Collagen metabolism in cultured adult rat cardiac fibroblasts:

response to angiotensin II and aldosterone. J Mol Cell Cardiol 1994;26:809–20.

[35] Kostuk WJ, Kazamias TM, Gander MP, et al. Left ventricular size after acute myocardial infarction. Serial changes and their prognostic significance. Circulation 1973;47:1174–9.

[36] Eaton LW, Weiss JL, Bulkley BH, et al. Regional cardiac dilatation after acute myocardial infarction: recognition by two-dimensional echocardiography. N Engl J Med 1979;300:57–62.

[37] Risk stratification and survival after myocardial infarction. N Engl J Med 1983;309:331–6.

[38] MacFadyen RJ, Barr CS, Struthers AD. Aldosterone blockade reduces vascular collagen turnover, improves heart rate variability and reduces early morning rise in heart rate in heart failure patients. Cardiovasc Res 1997;35:30–4.

[39] Rocha R, Rudolph AE, Frierdich GE, et al. Aldosterone induces a vascular inflammatory phenotype in the rat heart. Am J Physiol Heart Circ Physiol 2002;283:H1802–10.

[40] Wang W. Chronic administration of aldosterone depresses baroreceptor reflex function in the dog. Hypertension 1994;24:571–5.

[41] Yee KM, Struthers AD. Aldosterone blunts the baroreflex response in man. Clin Sci (Lond) 1998;95: 687–92.

[42] Barr CS, Lang CC, Hanson J, et al. Effects of adding spironolactone to an angiotensin-converting enzyme inhibitor in chronic congestive heart failure secondary to coronary artery disease. Am J Cardiol 1995; 76:1259–65.

[43] Yee KM, Pringle SD, Struthers AD. Circadian variation in the effects of aldosterone blockade on heart rate variability and QT dispersion in congestive heart failure. J Am Coll Cardiol 2001;37: 1800–7.

[44] Perrier R, Richard S, Sainte-Marie Y, et al. A direct relationship between plasma aldosterone and cardiac L-type Ca2+ current in mice. J Physiol 2005; 569:153–62.

[45] Schafer A, Fraccarollo D, Hildemann SK, et al. Addition of the selective aldosterone receptor antagonist eplerenone to ACE inhibition in heart failure: effect on endothelial dysfunction. Cardiovasc Res 2003;58:655–62.

[46] De Angelis N, Fiordaliso F, Latini R, et al. Appraisal of the role of angiotensin II and aldosterone in ventricular myocyte apoptosis in adult normotensive rat. J Mol Cell Cardiol 2002;34:1655–65.

[47] Biondi-Zoccai GG, Abbate A, Baldi A. Potential antiapoptotic activity of aldosterone antagonists in postinfarction remodeling. Circulation 2003;108: e26.

[48] Modena MG, Aveta P, Menozzi A, et al. Aldosterone inhibition limits collagen synthesis and progressive left ventricular enlargement after anterior myocardial infarction. Am Heart J 2001;141: 41–6.

[49] Di Pasquale P, Cannizzaro S, Giubilato A, et al. Additional beneficial effects of canrenoate in patients with anterior myocardial infarction on ACE-inhibitor treatment. A pilot study. Ital Heart J 2001;2: 121–9.

[50] Hayashi M, Tsutamoto T, Wada A, et al. Immediate administration of mineralocorticoid receptor antagonist spironolactone prevents post-infarct left ventricular remodeling associated with suppression of a marker of myocardial collagen synthesis in patients with first anterior acute myocardial infarction. Circulation 2003;107:2559–65.

[51] Pitt B, Remme W, Zannad F, et al. Eplerenone, a selective aldosterone blocker, in patients with left ventricular dysfunction after myocardial infarction. N Engl J Med 2003;348:1309–21.

[52] Aronson D, Rayfield EJ, Chesebro JH. Mechanisms determining course and outcome of diabetic patients who have had acute myocardial infarction. Ann Intern Med 1997;126:296–306.

[53] Pitt B, White H, Nicolau J, et al. Eplerenone reduces mortality 30 days after randomization following acute myocardial infarction in patients with left ventricular systolic dysfunction and heart failure. J Am Coll Cardiol 2005;46:425–31.

[54] Pitt B, Gheorghiade M, Zannad F, et al. Evaluation of eplerenone in the subgroup of EPHESUS patients with baseline left ventricular ejection fraction <or= 30%. Eur J Heart Fail 2006;8:295–301.

[55] Go AS, Chertow GM, Fan D, et al. Chronic kidney disease and the risks of death, cardiovascular events, and hospitalization. N Engl J Med 2004;351: 1296–305.

[56] Anavekar NS, McMurray JJ, Velazquez EJ, et al. Relation between renal dysfunction and cardiovascular outcomes after myocardial infarction. N Engl J Med 2004;351:1285–95.

[57] Ahmed A, Zannad F, Love TE, et al. A propensity-matched study of the association of low serum potassium levels and mortality in chronic heart failure. Eur Heart J 2007;28:1334–43.

[58] Pitt B, Zannad F, Remme WJ, et al. The effect of spironolactone on morbidity and mortality in patients with severe heart failure. Randomized Aldactone Evaluation Study Investigators. N Engl J Med 1999;341:709–17.

[59] Juurlink DN, Mamdani MM, Lee DS, et al. Rates of hyperkalemia after publication of the Randomized Aldactone Evaluation Study. N Engl J Med 2004; 351:543–51.

[60] Chakko SC, Frutchey J, Gheorghiade M. Life-threatening hyperkalemia in severe heart failure. Am Heart J 1989;117(5):1083–91.

[61] Anderson JL, Adams CD, Antman EM, et al. ACC/AHA 2007 Guidelines for the Management of Patients With Unstable Angina/Non ST-Elevation Myocardial Infarction. A Report of the American College of Cardiology/American Heart Association Task Force on Practice Guidelines (Writing

Committee to Revise the 2002 Guidelines for the Management of Patients With Unstable Angina/Non ST-Elevation Myocardial Infarction). Circulation 2007;116:e148–304.

[62] Freemantle N, Cleland J, Young P, et al. beta Blockade after myocardial infarction: systematic review and meta regression analysis. BMJ 1999;318:1730–7.

[63] Gottlieb SS, McCarter RJ, Vogel RA. Effect of beta-blockade on mortality among high-risk and low-risk patients after myocardial infarction. N Engl J Med 1998;339:489–97.

[64] Kober L, Torp-Pedersen C, Carlsen JE, et al. A clinical trial of the angiotensin-converting-enzyme inhibitor trandolapril in patients with left ventricular dysfunction after myocardial infarction. Trandolapril Cardiac Evaluation (TRACE) Study Group. N Engl J Med 1995;333:1670–6.

[65] Pfeffer MA, Braunwald E, Moye LA, et al. Effect of captopril on mortality and morbidity in patients with left ventricular dysfunction after myocardial infarction. Results of the survival and ventricular enlargement trial. The SAVE Investigators. N Engl J Med 1992;327:669–77.

[66] Effect of ramipril on mortality and morbidity of survivors of acute myocardial infarction with clinical evidence of heart failure. The Acute Infarction Ramipril Efficacy (AIRE) Study Investigators. Lancet 1993;342:821–8.

[67] Dickstein K, Kjekshus J. Effects of losartan and captopril on mortality and morbidity in high-risk patients after acute myocardial infarction: the OPTIMAAL randomised trial. Optimal Trial in Myocardial Infarction with Angiotensin II Antagonist Losartan. Lancet 2002;360:752–60.

[68] Randomised trial of cholesterol lowering in 4444 patients with coronary heart disease: the Scandinavian Simvastatin Survival Study (4S). Lancet 1994;344:1383–9.

[69] Sacks FM, Pfeffer MA, Moye LA, et al. CARE: the effect of pravastatin on coronary events after myocardial infarction in patients with average cholesterol levels. Cholesterol and Recurrent Events Trial investigators. N Engl J Med 1996;335:1001–9.

[70] Arntz HR, Agrawal R, Wunderlich W, et al. L-CAD: beneficial effects of pravastatin (+/-colestyramine/niacin) initiated immediately after a coronary event (the randomized Lipid-Coronary Artery Disease [L-CAD] Study). Am J Cardiol 2000;86:1293–8.

[71] Schwartz GG, Olsson AG, Ezekowitz MD, et al. MIRACL: effects of atorvastatin on early recurrent ischemic events in acute coronary syndromes: the MIRACL study: a randomized controlled trial. JAMA 2001;285:1711–8.

[72] Stenestrand U, Wallentin L. RIKS-HIA: early statin treatment following acute myocardial infarction and 1-year survival. JAMA 2001;285:430–6.

[73] Cannon CP, Braunwald E, McCabe CH, et al. PROVE IT-TIMI 22: intensive versus moderate lipid lowering with statins after acute coronary syndromes. N Engl J Med 2004;350:1495–504.

ELSEVIER
SAUNDERS

Cardiol Clin 26 (2008) 107–112

CARDIOLOGY
CLINICS

Differences in European and North American Approaches to the Management of Heart Failure

Philip A. Poole-Wilson, MB, MD, FRCP, FMedSci

Cardiac Medicine, National Heart & Lung Institute, Imperial College London, Dovehouse Street,
London SW3 6LY, UK

In the last few years there has been a proliferation of guidelines relating to the diagnosis, management and treatment of patients with all forms of heart failure. Three guidelines have been published from North America, namely those of the Heart Failure Society of America [1], the American Heart Association [2], and the Canadian Heart Association [3]. Europe has guidelines from the European Society of Cardiology [4,5], from SIGN in Scotland (Scottish Intercollegiate Guidelines Network) [6] and from NICE (National Institute for Clinical Excellence) in the United Kingdom [7]. Guidelines have also been published in Australia [8]. In general there are no great differences between the guidelines. Those only emerge on inspection of the details in some controversial topics in the treatment of heart failure.

There are many reasons for making guidelines available. These extend from providing information and advice to doctors and health carers, the delivery of best care according to protocols, promoting equality and equity for the provision of health care across a country, the need to ensure the use of effective drugs or devices, the need to ensure safety, the need to control the costs of health provision, and ultimately to the audit of that health provision. These are noble objectives but often the allegation is made that a primary determinant of guidelines is the control of costs. There is certainly some truth in that argument. Governments would not wish to encourage the use of highly expensive treatments where a small benefit is acquired at a vast cost to the detriment of the availability and quality of treatments provided to other groups of patients with other diseases.

E-mail address: p.poole-wilson@imperial.ac.uk

Cost control is closely related to the system of health provision in a country so that subtle differences exist between procedures in the United States and in Europe. The FDA (Federal Drug Agency) is the major body controlling the use of drugs and devices in medicine in the United States. It is concerned with efficacy and safety but increasingly with the issue of how medical practice should be conducted. In Europe the key body is the MHRA (Medical Healthcare products Regulatory Agency) which in general is limited to determining the effectiveness and risks of treatments. With devices the appropriate agency is only concerned with whether the device functions as it is proposed, not with the issue of whether it is effective in clinical practice. Clinical practice in Europe is increasingly determined by guidelines and by bodies such as NICE. NICE is a body in the UK, independent of the government, which makes judgements as to whether the use of a drug or device is sufficiently cost effective to merit a recommendation that it be used across the country. Other countries in Europe have slightly different procedures but in general there is separation between those bodies which determine risk and benefit and those which assess how a treatment should be used within a country.

Several recent studies have demonstrated unequivocally that adherence to guidelines and attention to treatment improves outcomes in the treatment of heart failure [9–11]. The improvement can be as a reduction in mortality in absolute terms of as much as 10 deaths per 100 patients years over a period of 3 years. Nevertheless there are many limitations to guidelines. Guidelines are not infallible, do not overrule clinical judgement and should be regarded as guidelines not directives.

Process for guidelines and grading systems

The credibility of guidelines is heavily dependent on the reviewing process [12–14]. The purpose is to avoid bias or influence form individual opinions and financial influence. In guidelines on specialist topics, such as heart failure, that leads to an impasse. The influence of experts in a topic (eg, electrophysiology and implantable cardioverter defibrillators (ICDs)), general cardiologists with an interest in heart failure, and general physicians, health care specialists and those responsible for the delivery of health care will vary. All have biases and conflicts of interest declared or not. Most guidelines give ultimate authority to groups made up from generalists and insist on declarations of any perceived or possible conflict of interests. But there is little evidence that such a system is effective and it is difficult to comprehend how a health provider can comment on the nuances of, say, electrophysiology in other than a superficial manner. The problem remains unresolved.

Guidelines often choose to grade their opinions on the value of treatments. Many systems are used and these often conflict (Tables 1–6) [6,7,15–17]. Most physicians almost certainly do not know what a grade of 2 B means. Furthermore there are different meanings assigned to the same numbers and letters. Confusion arises when numbers or alphabetical letters are used for the type of evidence, the quality of the source of evidence and the recommendation. Data derived from observational

Table 1
ACC/AHA grading for recommendations in guidelines

Classes		Levels of evidence	
I	Intervention is useful and effective	A	Data derived from multiple randomized clinical trials
IIA	Evidence conflicts / opinions differ, but leans toward efficacy	B	Data derived from a single RCT or non-randomized studies
IIB	Evidence conflicts / opinions differ, but leans against efficacy	C	Consensus opinion of experts
III	Intervention is not useful or effective and may be harmful		

Data from Gibbons RJ, Abrams J, Chatterjee K, et al. ACC/AHA 2002 guideline update for the management of patients with chronic stable angina—summary article: a report of the American College of Cardiology/American Heart Association Task Force on Practice Guidelines (Committee on the Management of Patients With Chronic Stable Angina). J Am Coll Cardiol 2003;41:159–68.

Table 2
Grading for recommendations in guidelines

Class I	Benefit > > > Risk Procedure or treatment SHOULD be performed or administered
Class IIa	Benefit > > Risk Additional studies with focused objectives needed IT IS REASONABLE to perform procedure or administer treatment
Class IIb	Benefit ≥ Risk Additional studies with broad objectives needed; Additional registry data would be helpful Procedure or treatment MAY BE CONSIDERED

Data from Smith SC, Allen J, Blair SN, et al. AHA/ACC guidelines for secondary prevention for patients with coronary and other atherosclerotic vascular disease: 2006 update. J Am Coll Cardiol 2006;47:2130–9.

studies and registries is of substantially less value than that from well conducted clinical trials. In cardiology so many large trials have refuted the strongly held views of clinicians based on observational data. There is a strong argument for simplification and uniformity of these classifications so that understandable recommendations are made in clearer language which can be understood across the world.

Selected limitations of guidelines on heart failure

A critical and important limitation of many guidelines is the nature of the evidence on which guidelines are based. This problem is particularly prominent in relation to heart failure where there is a large database but the application to the whole community is questionable. In the general population the mean age of persons with heart failure is 75 years and the overall prevalence is the same in males and females. In clinical trials the mean age is in the low 60s and often only 25% of patients are female. There is a lack of data on the benefit and risk of management strategies in the elderly, in females and in ethnic groups.

The guidelines from both Europe and the US use the exact inclusion criteria and the treatment strategies in trials to formulate their recommendations. That can be misleading. For example the recommendations for the use of ICDs and cardiac resynchronisation therapy (CRT) suggest use of these devices in patients where the ejection fraction is below 30 and 35%. The mean ejection fraction in the two relevant trials [18,19] was 23 and 25%. Thus the recommendation is based on the inclusion criteria and not the actual population recruited into the trial. In these two examples

Table 3
Grading for recommendations in guidelines

A hierarchy of evidence		Typical grading of recommendations	
Level	Type of evidence	Grade	Evidence
1a	Evidence obtained from systematic review of meta-analysis of randomized controlled trials	A	At least one randomized controlled trial as part of a body of literature of overall good quality and consistency addressing the specific recommendation (evidence levels 1a and 1b)
1b	Evidence obtained from at least one randomized controlled trial		
IIa	Evidence obtained from at least one well designed controlled study without randomization	B	Well-conducted clinical studies but no randomized clinical trials on the topics of recommendation (evidence levels IIa, IIb and III)
IIb	Evidence obtained from at least one other type of well-designed quasi-experimental study	C	Expert committee reports or opinions and/or clinical experience of respected authorities. This grading indicates that directly applicable clinical studies of good quality are absent (evidence level IV)
III	Evidence obtained from well-designed non-experimental descriptive studies, such as comparative studies, correlation studies and case studies		
IV	Evidence obtained from expert committee reports or opinions and/or clinical experience of respected authorities	GPP	Recommended good practice based on the clinical experience of the Guideline Development Group
DS	Diagnostic studies	DS	Diagnostic studies
NICE	Evidence from NICE guidelines or health technology appraisal program	NICE	Evidence from NICE guidelines or health technology appraisal program

From National Collaborating Center for Chronic Conditions. Chronic heart failure: national clinical guideline for diagnosis and management in primary and secondary care. London: Royal College of Physicians, 2003. Copyright © 2003, Royal College of Physicians. Reproduced by permission..

Table 4
Grading for recommendations in guidelines

Statements of evidence	
Ia	Evidence obtained from meta-analysis of randomized controlled trials.
Ib	Evidence obtained from at least one randomized controlled trial.
IIa	Evidence obtained from at least one well-designed controlled study without randomization.
IIb	Evidence obtained from at least one other type of well-designed quasiexperimental study.
III	Evidence obtained from well-designed non-experimental descriptive studies, such as comparative studies, correlation studies and case studies.
IV	Evidence obtained from expert committee reports or opinions and/or clinical experiences of respected authorities.
Grades of recommendations	
A	Requires at least one randomized controlled trial as part of a body of literature of overall good quality and consistency addressing the specific recommendation. (Evidence levels Ia, Ib)
B	Requires the availability of well conducted clinical studies but no randomized clinical trials on the topic of recommendation. (Evidence levels IIa, IIb, III)
C	Requires evidence obtained from expert committee reports or opinions and/or clinical experiences of respected authorities. Indicates an absence of directly applicable clinical studies of good quality. (Evidence level IV)

SIGN Guideline No 35 1999.

Table 5
Different meanings of class 1 grading

Intervention is useful and effective ACC/AHA Gibbons RJ, et al. J Am Coll Cardiol 2003;41:159–68.	
Evidence and/or general agreement that a given diagnostic procedure/treatment is beneficial, useful and effective The Task Force on Acute Heart Failure Eur Heart J 2005;26:384–416.	
1a	Evidence obtained from systematic review of meta-analysis of randomized controlled trials
1b	Evidence obtained from at least one randomized controlled trial NICE guideline number 5 Chronic Heart Failure 2006
Benefit > > > Risk.	
Procedure or treatment SHOULD be performed or administered ACC/AHA. Circulation 2006;113: 2363–72.	

the difference is so large as to make the recommendations unreasonable.

A further problem is the wording of recommendations. Some recommendations use words such as "consider." A hedging word, and consequently carry little authority. Alternatively recommendations use words such as "must" or "should." Such

Table 6
A possible solution to the problem of grading

Evidence grade	Interpretation of evidence
I: High.	Research provides robust and accurate information about treatment, diagnosis or prognosis.
II: Intermediate.	Limitations in research mean there is some uncertainty about findings.
III: Low.	ubstantial limitations in research mean that findings cannot be considered robust.
Recommendation grade	Interpretation of recommendation
A	Recommendation. There is clear evidence to recommend a pattern of care
B	Provisional recommendation On balance a pattern of care is recommended although there are uncertainties
C	Consensus opinion The group recommends a pattern of care based on its shared understanding

Nice Guidelines August 2004.

absolute positions have no place in medicine and are will be misleading to the lay public or to uninformed health providers. An example is the statement "Angiotensin-converting enzyme (ACE) inhibitors are recommended as first-line therapy in patients with a reduced left ventricular systolic function ...... with or without symptoms (Class of recommendation I, level of evidence A)" [5]. This statement could be thought to indicate all such patients must receive this treatment and that the treatment is given to all these patients before the use of a diuretic.

Major differences between American and European guidelines

These are few, probably because the writers are familiar with each the opinions of others and writers are reviewing the same databases. There are differences in the grading of some treatments but that is largely explained by the different criteria applied. Currently one of the key differences is in the semantics of heart failure. The adjectives acute, advanced and decompensated are often used almost interchangeably and this leads to confusion in the interpretation of trials because it is not clear just what is the phenotype of patients included in studies. This is particularly true for the phrase acute heart failure (Table 7) [2,4]. In many countries of the world this phrase was (is) used to identify patients who have acute pulmonary edema, a medical emergency because of impending death of the patient. The emphasis was on the severity of the illness. More recent definitions are rather vague (see Table 7) but appear to refer to new onset heart failure and admission to hospital. The word "rapid" is contained in both definitions but remains undefined and could mean hours, days or even a week or two. The problem nccds rcsolution with more careful and precise descriptions of the phenotype.

Table 7
Different definitions of acute heart failure syndromes

AHFS is characterized by a rapid or gradual onset of signs and symptoms of heart failure, resulting in unplanned hospitalizations or office or emergency room visits.	AHA/ACCguidelines
AHF is defined as the rapid onset of symptoms and signs, secondary to abnormal cardiac function	ESC guidelines 2005

Specific differences between guidelines

In general agreement is more prominent than differences in the treatment of heart faiure. There is unanimity that the routine treatment of heart failure is diuretics to control fluid overload, angiotensin converting enzyme (ACE) inhibitors and beta-blockers. In those patients who do not tolerate an ACE inhibitor an angiotensin receptor blocker (ARB) is appropriate and in severe heart failure an aldosterone inhibitor can be added. There are differences in the grading for the many other options in the treatment of heart failure. In the opinion of this author the grading system is flawed and not suitable to specify just how such treatments should be used in clinical practice and it would be preferable to state uncertainty where it exists and the indications where such treatments may be helpful to the patient. Absolute statements on for example the use of anti-arrhythmic drugs, pacemakers, ICDs, CRT, devices and transplantation should be avoided.

There are two differences which could matter. The European guidelines all advise the use of the measurement of brain natriuretic peptide (BNP) as a screening test before proceeding to an echocardiogram whereas the US guideline simply recommends an echocardiogram in any patient thought to have heart failure and puts less reliance on the measurement of BNP. The Australian guideline [8] takes the same position. In reality on both continents the echocardiogram is regarded as the key imaging modality and, in the opinion of many, should be undertaken in almost all patients with suspected heart failure regardless of the BNP. The recommendation is not aimed at large secondary or tertiary hospitals to which highly selected groups of patient are referred. Rather the advice is aimed at a general approach to the problem of heart failure in the community as a whole.

A second difference is the emphasis given to the use of diuretics. The European guidelines [5] in the text on pharmacologic treatment place diuretics uncomfortably between ACE inhibitors and beta-blockers. The guideline states "There are no controlled randomized trials that have assessed the effect on symptoms or survival of these agents. Diuretics should always be administered in combination with ACE-inhibitors and beta-blockers if tolerated (Class of recommendation I, level of evidence C)." The first sentence is probably untrue [20]. The second sentence makes an absolute statement about what is not usual practice. This could easily be misunderstood by

Table 8
Barriers to the successful implementation of guidelines

Health care systems	Physicians	Patients
Organizational constraints	Lack of awareness, familiarity, and agreement	Lack of awareness and understanding
Lack of reimbursement	Low motivation and/or outcome expectancy	Limited access to care
Inadequate staffing resource and specialist support	Inability to reconcile guidelines with patient preferences	Low level of compliance; reluctance to take life-long medication
Increased liability	Insufficient time and/or resource	Lack of adherence to lifestyle modifications

Data from Erhardt L. Barriers to effective implementation of guideline recommendations. Am J Med 2005;118 suppl 12A:36–41 and Cabana MD, Rand CS, Powe NR, et al. Why don't physicians follow clinical practice guidelines? A framework for improvement. JAMA 1999;282:1458–65.

non-medical personnel. Often a patient presenting with heart failure and shortness of breath will be treated with a diuretic and the use of an ACE inhibitor introduced only after the results of biochemical measurements are known, The SIGN guidelines place the diuretic group of drugs fourth behind all the other conventional groups of drugs. The HFSA do much the same. Only the AHA/ACC [2] guideline puts diuretics as the first line of treatment in patients with systolic heart failure and symptoms; and they are probably right.

Rather than continue to mull over minor differences between guidelines, the time has come for more attention to be directed toward the implementation of what we know and is stated in guidelines. In that way more will be achieved for the health of patients with heart failure (Table 8) [21,22].

Summary

Guidelines for heart failure are many. The consistency of the recommendations far exceeds any differences. Guidelines would be improved if there were greater clarity of intent on some topics and the current grading systems abandoned. Where the data is conflicting or no consensus of opinion exists, that should be stated. Guidelines are often used for audit and to provide appropriate care by health care specialists. For that reason guidelines must give simple direction to standard medical practice in language which cannot be misunderstood.

References

[1] Executive summary: HFSA 2006 Comprehensive Heart Failure Practice Guideline. J Card Fail 2006; 12:10–38.

[2] Hunt SA, Abraham WT, Chin MH, et al. ACC/ AHA 2005 Guideline Update for the Diagnosis and Management of Chronic Heart Failure in the Adult: a report of the American College of Cardiology/American Heart Association Task Force on Practice Guidelines (Writing Committee to Update the 2001 Guidelines for the Evaluation and Management of Heart Failure): developed in collaboration with the American College of Chest Physicians and the International Society for Heart and Lung Transplantation: endorsed by the Heart Rhythm Society. Circulation 2005;112:E154–235.

[3] Arnold JM, Howlett JG, Dorian P, et al. Canadian Cardiovascular Society Consensus Conference recommendations on heart failure update 2007: Prevention, management during intercurrent illness or acute decompensation, and use of biomarkers. Can J Cardiol 2007;23:21–45.

[4] Nieminen MS, Bohm M, Cowie MR, et al. Executive summary of the guidelines on the diagnosis and treatment of acute heart failure: the Task Force on acute heart failure of the European Society of Cardiology. Eur Heart J 2005;26:384–416.

[5] Swedberg K, Cleland J, Dargie H, et al. Guidelines for the diagnosis and treatment of chronic heart failure: executive summary (update 2005): the Task Force for the diagnosis and treatment of chronic heart failure of the European Society of Cardiology. Eur Heart J 2005;26:1115–40.

[6] SIGN. Scottish Intercollegiate Guidelines Network. 95 Management of chronic heart failure. A national clinical guideline. Available at: www.sign.ac.uk. 1–55. 2007. Accessed February 6, 2007.

[7] Guideline Development Group. NICE Guidelines. Developed by The National Collaborating Centre for Chronic Conditions. Chronic heart failure. National clinical guidelines for diagnosis and management in primary and secondary care NICE guideline No. 5. London: Royal College of Physicians; 2003. p. 1–163.

[8] Krum H, Jelinek MV, Stewart S, et al. Guidelines for the prevention, detection and management of people with chronic heart failure in Australia 2006. Med J Aust 2006;185:549–57.

[9] Komajda M, Lapuerta P, Hermans N, et al. Adherence to guidelines is a predictor of outcome in chronic heart failure: the MAHLER survey. Eur Heart J 2005;26:1653–9.

[10] Cleland JG, Louis AA, Rigby AS, et al. Noninvasive home telemonitoring for patients with heart failure at high risk of recurrent admission and death: the Trans-European Network-Home-Care Management System (TEN-HMS) study. J Am Coll Cardiol 2005;45:1654–64.

[11] Opasich C, Boccanelli A, Cafiero M, et al. Programme to improve the use of beta-blockers for heart failure in the elderly and in those with severe symptoms: results of the BRING-UP 2 Study. Eur J Heart Fail 2006;8:649–57.

[12] Burgers JS, Cluzeau FA, Hanna SE, et al. Characteristics of high-quality guidelines: evaluation of 86 clinical guidelines developed in ten European countries and Canada. Int J Technol Assess Health Care 2003;19:148–57.

[13] Minhas R. Eminence-based guidelines: a quality assessment of the second Joint British Societies' guidelines on the prevention of cardiovascular disease. Int J Clin Pract 2007;61:1137–44.

[14] AGREE Collaboration. Development and validation of an international appraisal instrument for assessing the quality of clinical practice guidelines: the AGREE project. Qual Saf Health Care 2003;12:18–23.

[15] Gibbons RJ, Abrams J, Chatterjee K, et al. ACC/ AHA 2002 guideline update for the management of patients with chronic stable angina–summary article: a report of the American College of Cardiology/American Heart Association Task Force on practice guidelines (Committee on the Management of Patients With Chronic Stable Angina). J Am Coll Cardiol 2003;41:159–68.

[16] Smith SC Jr, Allen J, Blair SN, et al. AHA/ACC guidelines for secondary prevention for patients with coronary and other atherosclerotic vascular disease: 2006 update: endorsed by the National Heart, Lung, and Blood Institute. Circulation 2006;113:2363–72.

[17] North of England Hypertension Guideline Developmetn Group (NICE). Essential hypertension: managing adult patients in prinmarycare. Centre forf Health Services Reseach Report No 111. 1–261. 2004.

[18] Moss AJ, Zareba W, Hall WJ, et al. Prophylactic implantation of a defibrillator in patients with myocardial infarction and reduced ejection fraction. N Engl J Med 2002;346:877–83.

[19] Cleland JG, Daubert JC, Erdmann E, et al. The effect of cardiac resynchronization on morbidity and mortality in heart failure. N Engl J Med 2005; 352:1539–49.

[20] Faris R, Flather MD, Purcell H, et al. Diuretics for heart failure. Cochrane Database Syst Rev 2006; CD003838.

[21] Cabana MD, Rand CS, Powe NR, et al. Why don't physicians follow clinical practice guidelines? A framework for improvement. JAMA 1999;282:1458–65.

[22] Erhardt LR. Barriers to effective implementation of guideline recommendations. Am J Med 2005; 118(Suppl 12A):36–41.

ELSEVIER
SAUNDERS

Cardiol Clin 26 (2008) 113–125

CARDIOLOGY
CLINICS

Heart Failure: Who We Treat Versus Who We Study

Leslie W. Miller, MD

Washington Hospital Center and Georgetown University, 110 Irving Street NW, 1E-7, Washington, DC 20010, USA

The prevalence of patients with the diagnosis of heart failure (HF) continues to increase, with recent data suggesting that the current estimate in the United States should now be over 7 million patients. This estimate is based on the recent census confirming a current population of 300 million people in the United States, and an estimated average prevalence of heart failure in 2.5% of the population [1–4]. There are many sources of information about the patients with heart failure, including population surveys [5–14] and data from patients identified and followed from the time of a hospitalization for HF [15–17], as well as inpatient registries [18,19]. Many patients have been enrolled in pharmaceutical and devices trials in HF, but the patients enrolled are often not reflective of the patients being managed outside of these trials in terms of age, gender, race, and comorbidities. And yet, investigators have extrapolated the results of these trials to all patients with heart failure. This article is a comparison of the demographics and outcomes of the patients with heart failure that are treated and those that have been studied.

Age

There are many demographic factors that influence the prevalence of HF, but age is the most powerful influence. It is clear that heart failure is a disease of advancing age, being relatively uncommon in those below the age of 50 years, but the disease increases progressively with each subsequent decade [1–4]. It affects as many as 10% to 15% of people over the age of

65 years, and even higher in those over 75 years (Fig. 1). The average age of patients admitted to the hospital is 75 years [2–19]. Patients over 65 years make up only 12% of the population, but account for 38% of hospital discharges and 46% of hospital days [2]. The finding of preponderance of hospitalized patients being elderly is also reflected in data from the Centers for Disease Control [2], which showed almost no increase in the number of patients under the age of 64 years who were hospitalized with HF over the last 25 years, while the number between 64 and 84 years, and those over the age of 85 years, has nearly doubled (Fig. 2). The population over 65 years is expected to double in the next 20 years from an estimated 32 million in the year 2000, to nearly 70 million by the year 2025 [2,3]. Thus, heart failure will be a major health problem for the aging United States population for the next several decades.

Race and gender

The prevalence of heart failure varies considerably by race and gender [20–26]. Data have shown that the overall prevalence is essentially equal between men and women, averaging approximately 2.4% in males and 2.6% in females [1–4]. However, this percentage varies between 2.5% and 3.1% in males, being highest in African American males, and between 1.6% and 3.5% in females, with the lowest prevalence in Latino women and highest in African American women (Table 1). More men seem to have HF under the age of 55 years, but women are equally affected thereafter, and by living an average of 7 years longer, women have an equal overall prevalence. The percentage of men who are hospitalized is nearly equal, as shown in

E-mail address: leslie.w.miller@medstar.net

0733-8651/08/$ - see front matter © 2008 Elsevier Inc. All rights reserved.
doi:10.1016/j.ccl.2007.10.005

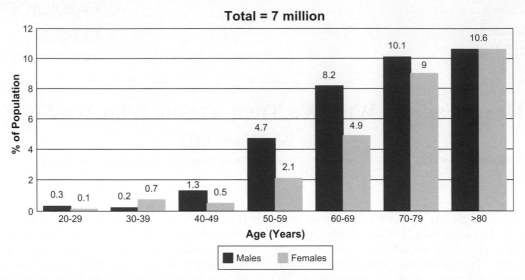

Fig. 1. Impact of age and gender on the prevalence of heart failure. (*Data from* Thom T, Haase N, Rosamond W, et al. Heart disease and stroke statistics—2006 update: A report from the American Heart Association Statistics Committee and Stroke Statistics Subcommittee. Circulation. 2006;113:e85-e151.)

the large Acute Decompensated Heart Failure National Registry (ADHERE) database [19,20]. The racial mix was predominantly Caucasian, but reflective of national race percentages and disease prevalence. The mortality also varies considerably by race and gender, with the highest mortality of 3.5% in African American females.

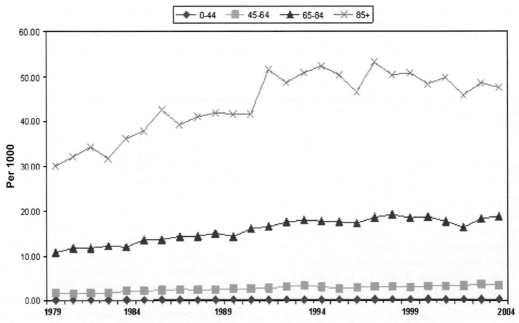

Fig. 2. Influence of age on the rate of hospitalization for heart failure. (*From* Centers for Disease Control. Heart failure fact sheet. Atlanta, GA: Centers for Disease Control and Prevention, 2006. Available at http://www.cdc.gov/dhdsp/library/pdfs/fs_heart_failure.pdf.)

Table 1
Differing prevalence and incidence of heart failure by race and gender

Population	Prevalence	New cases	Mortality	Hosp D/Cs
Total	7 M	500,000	57,000 (287K)	1.1 M
Males	2.4 M (2.6%)		22,300 (39%)	
Females	2.6 M (2.1%)		34,905 (61%)	
NHW males	2.5%			
NHW females	1.9%			
AA males	3.1%			
AA females	3.5%			
Latino males	2.7%			
Latino females	1.6%			

Abbreviations: AA, African American; D/Cs, discharges; M, million; NHW, nonwhite hispanic.

Data from Heart Disease and Stroke Statistics—2006 Update. A Report from the American Heart Association Statistics Committee and Stroke Statistics Subcommittee. Circulation. 2006;113:e85–151. Available at: http://circ.ahajournals.org/cgi/content/full/113/6/e85#TBL9.

Etiology and type of heart failure

It is clear that there are significant differences in both the etiology and type of heart failure by race, gender, and age. African Americans typically have hypertension as the major cause of their HF, while ischemic heart disease is the primary cause in Caucasians [1–4]. African Americans present typically at a younger age than Caucasians, with more advance heart failure at presentation, have a 3- to 7-fold higher incidence of hypertension as the cause of HF, and a 15- to 18-fold higher incidence of end stage renal disease compared with Caucasians.

Recently it has also become clear that a nearly equal percentage of patients with heart failure have preserved systolic function (formerly called diastolic heart failure) as have reduced systolic function, in both the United States [27–32] and Europe [33,34]. The ADHERE database [19] showed that 46% of patients hospitalized had an ejection fraction (EF) greater than 40% by echocardiography. There are several differences in the demographics of those with preserved versus reduced systolic function, as noted in Table 2. It is clear that the prevalence of heart failure with preserved systolic function increases significantly with advancing age, and is much more common in women and those with a history of hypertension.

The much higher prevalence of heart failure with preserved systolic function in women was demonstrated in a study by Vasan and colleagues [29] conducted from the Framingham database. These investigators performed an echocardiogram on a random sample of 74 patients being followed for heart failure by their criteria. The data showed that over 50% of men in the random sample had an EF greater than 41% and nearly 30% had an EF greater than 50%. In comparison, of the 33 women in this study, 80% had an EF greater than 41%, and 75% had an EF greater than 50%. In contrast, the incidence of coronary artery disease is lower in those with preserved EF, compared with those with reduced EF (52.9% versus 63.7%). There are also differences in comorbidities between patients with preserved versus reduced systolic function, including the incidence of atrial fibrillation, which is more common in those with preserved EF (41% versus 28%) [27,28,31].

Comorbidities

Patients with HF often have a number of comorbidities. Several databases have shown that there is a very high prevalence of diabetes in patients with heart failure, averaging as much as 40% [35–39]. While the majority of patients with diabetes will develop atherosclerosis and coronary artery disease as the cause of their heart failure, patients with diabetes who do not have coronary artery disease may have an even higher mortality than those with coronary artery disease [7]. Hypertension is the primary cause of HF in the African American patients, but is also common in other racial groups and significantly predisposes patients to the development of HF. Patients with ischemic etiology of their heart failure often have hyperlipidemia, and an increasing percentage of HF patients are obese [1–4]. Recent data have suggested however, that there is a surprising paradox of increased survival in obese patients with HF [40]. Renal dysfunction is

Table 2

Clinical demographics of patients with heart failure and either preserved or reduced ejection fraction

Characteristic	Reduced EF	Preserved EF	P value
Age	71.7	74.4	<0.001
Male sex (%)	65.4	44.3	0.17
BMI	28.6	29.7	0.002
Obesity	35.5	41.4	0.007
Serum creatinine	1.6 ± 1.0	1.6 ± 1.1	NS
Hypertension	48.0	62.7	<0.001
CAD	63.7	52.9	<0.001
Diabetes	34.3	33.1	0.61
A Fib	28.5	41.3	<0.001

Abbreviations: A fib, atrial fibrillation; BMI, body mass index; CAD, coronary artery disease.

Data from Owan TE, Hodge DO, Herges RM, et al. Trends in prevalence and outcome of heart failure with preserved ejection fraction. N Engl J Medicine 2006;355(3):251–9.

becoming an increasing problem in patients with HF [41–48] and is caused by multiple factors, including advancing age and the coexistence of intrinsic renal disease secondary to hypertension or diabetes, as well as low perfusion and use of high doses of diuretics [48] and potentially nephrotoxic drugs, such as angiotensin-converting enzyme (ACE) inhibitors. The development of significant renal impairment has been shown to be a high risk factor for mortality, and has been confirmed in studies of both outpatient and hospitalized cohorts [42,47].

Survival

The survival with heart failure over the last decade has been variably reported [49,50], but several reports suggest that the survival has unfortunately declined over the last 15 years. The Framingham database [6] suggested that the average survival at 5 years, for all patients followed from the time of diagnosis of HF, was 50%. However, Owan and colleagues [27], from the Mayo Clinic, followed a large number of patients from Olmstead County, Minnesota over a 15-year period. Their data demonstrated that there had been approximately an 8% overall improvement in survival in those with systolic heart failure between 1987 and 2001, but in the most recent era survival was only 40% at 5 years. In contrast, there was no improvement in 5-year survival in patients with preserved systolic function and

symptomatic heart failure over this 15-year observation period, and a similar 40% survival at 5 years for those with preserved systolic function (Fig. 3), making it worse than most forms of cancer [51,52]. More recently, in a study of 2,445 patients with an average age of 76 years who were hospitalized in Worcester, Massachusetts for HF in the year 2000, and followed until 2005, showed that the all cause mortality at one year was 37%, and the survival at 5 years was only 21% [53]. The survival was lower in those whose first hospitalization for HF was the incident admission in the study.

Who investigators study

There are significant differences in the outcomes and demographics of those treated versus those studied in clinical trials [54–56]. This is a result of many factors, including the desire to avoid enrolling patients with comorbidities, such as renal insufficiency and other conditions that might adversely influence the outcome of trials independent of a treatment effect [57]. Therefore, investigators base nearly all of their current recommendations for the treatment of patients with heart failure on clinical trials which have had a disproportionately small percentage of those with the highest prevalence of the disease.

Survival

The body of evidence of results in HF trials is nicely summarized in recently published HF guidelines [58,59]. The survival of patients with HF in clinical studies is often much better than what has been reported in population studies described above. There is a uniform finding that survival worsens with advancing stage of the disease, but there is a great deal of variability in the definition of Stage C HF, as evidence by recently published trials which reported 1-year mortalities that range from 11% to 35% [60–69], versus 37% to 57% in population studies. There is more uniformity of the data in those with the most advanced or refractory HF Stage D who have an extremely high mortality, which may be as high as 80% at 1 year [70,71].

Age

Although it has been shown that the prevalence of HF rises significantly over the age of 60 years, only a few studies have examined patients above this age. Heiat and Krumholz [55]

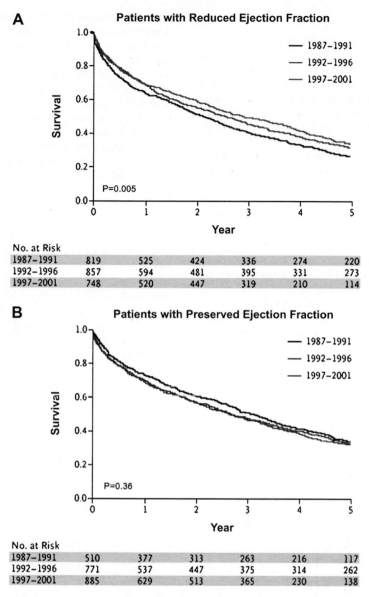

A **Patients with Reduced Ejection Fraction**

No. at Risk						
1987–1991	819	525	424	336	274	220
1992–1996	857	594	481	395	331	273
1997–2001	748	520	447	319	210	114

B **Patients with Preserved Ejection Fraction**

No. at Risk						
1987–1991	510	377	313	263	216	117
1992–1996	771	537	447	375	314	262
1997–2001	885	629	513	365	230	138

Fig. 3. Survival in patients with heart failure with either reduced (*A*) or preserved (*B*) systolic dysfunction over a 15-year period. *Reproduced from* Owan TE, Hodge DO, Herges RM, et al. Trends in prevalence and outcome of heart failure with preserved ejection fraction. N Engl J Medicine 2006;355(3):251–9; with permission.

examined the mean age of patients involved in heart failure studies and found that it averaged 59 years in the late 1980s, but rose to an average of 64 years in the late 1990s, largely because of a few studies specifically targeting older patients, such as the two evaluation of Losartan in the elderly trials [63], and the Heart Outcomes Prevention Evaluation [64]. The latter enrolled over 10,000 patients with an average age of 72 years. Subsequent trials, such as Candesartan in Heart Failure Assessment of Reduction in Mortality and Morbidity [65], had an average age of 66 years, but the very recent African American Heart Failure (AHFT) trial [60] had an average age of only 58 years. The ability of older patients to tolerate multiple drug regimens, and the doses used in these trials, is typically much less [72,73]. More studies are needed in the older population to verify the benefit and tolerability of HF medications reported in younger patients.

Race

Similar disparities exist by race, in particular lower percentages of African Americans and Latinos compared with Caucasians included in clinical trials [55]. Data show that until the last 2 to 3 years, there has been a disproportionately low percentage of nonwhites in heart failure trials, from a low of 13% in the late 1990s, to 27% in more recent studies, and the AHFT trial [60] conducted solely in African Americans. There have been very few Latino patients enrolled in any heart failure trials to date.

Does the lack of a broad representation of all subgroups with HF in most of the seminal trials upon which we have based our recommendations for therapy have any impact? The answer is, yes. Based on our understanding of the pathogenesis of heart failure, in particular the importance of the neurohormonal system, we have assumed that observations made in trials in which there were on average only 10% to 15% African Americans would hold in that population as well. However, this assumption has been shown to be quite erroneous, as shown in the meta-analysis by Shekelle and colleagues [74]. The reviews of the original studies of left ventricular dysfunction (SOLVD) prevention trial [75] for example demonstrated that there was a very substantial difference in the development of heart failure in African

Americans compared with Caucasians [76,77]. At 4 years of follow-up, 50% of the African Americans had developed symptomatic heart failure versus only 25% of the Caucasians (Fig. 4). Reanalysis of the data by race in the SOLVD treatment study [76] found no measurable difference in all cause or cardiovascular mortality by race, but there was a highly significant reduction in hospitalization for heart failure in Caucasians versus African Americans (0.54% versus 0.95%, $P = .005\%$). When death or hospitalization for heart failure were combined, there was also a significantly lower benefit, 9% in African Americans versus 25% in the Caucasian population ($P = .02$).

When beta-blocker trials were examined, Shekelle and colleagues [74] found that Caucasians have always benefited in the series of beta-blocker trials, including the beta-blocker evaluation of survival trial (BEST) [66], the Carvedilol prospective randomized cumulative survival trial [61], the Metoprolol CR/XL randomized intervention trail [65], and the United States Carvedilol trial [62], but African Americans represented less than 15% of those enrolled. When the benefit of Bisoprolol was examined retrospectively in the BEST trial [66], which had 27% African Americans, there was in fact an adverse affect of the beta blocker in the African Americans, compared

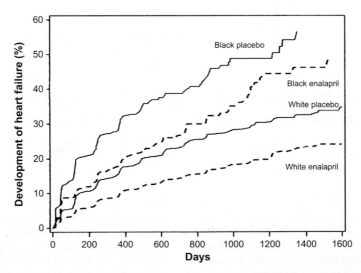

Fig. 4. Differing likelihood of development of heart failure by race in the SOLVD prevention trial of ACE inhibitors versus placebo in asymptomatic patients with reduced systolic function. *Reproduced from* Dries DL, Strong MH, Cooper RS, et al. Efficacy of angiotensin-converting enzyme inhibition in reducing progression from asymptomatic left ventricular dysfunction to symptomatic heart failure in black and white patients. J Am Coll Cardiol 2002;40(2):311–7; with permission.

with the Caucasians in the study, that nearly reached statistical significance. When these four trials were compared, there was no net benefit of beta-blockers in African Americans compared with the average 31% reduction in mortality in Caucasians.

The trial that had perhaps the greatest impact of race on outcome was the original vasodilator heart failure (VHFT-1) trial [78], which was conducted in Veterans Administration Hospitals with largely Caucasian males of an average age of 62 years. This trial was the first to show a survival advantage of the combination of hydralazine and nitrates, compared with prazosin or placebo (Fig. 5). When the data from that landmark study was examined retrospectively, it showed an insignificant difference in mortality in the Caucasian patients who received hydralazine throughout the 5-year follow-up, compared with a 47% relative risk reduction in African Americans (P = .04) [55]. This observation led to the AHFT trail [60] conducted exclusively among African Americans, which examined the benefit of adding hydralazine and nitrates versus placebo to the standard background combination of an ACE inhibitor, digoxin, and diuretics. The study was stopped prematurely because of a 43% relative risk reduction at 600 days in favor of the hydralazine-nitrate combination (Fig. 6). The findings have led to research which has demonstated a reduction in the production of nitric oxide in African Americans, who therefore, not surprisingly, benefited from the use of the antioxidant and

nitrate donor drug combination [78]. There are likely polymorphisms of multiple genes which are important in patients with heart failure, which provide some scientific basis for the disparities observed.

Gender

Another very substantial disparity has been the incredibly low percentage of women who have participated in cardiovascular trials of any type. Despite the equal prevalence of HF in women compared with men, the percentage of women who have been enrolled in HF trials since 1985 has averaged only 22% [55]. Many of the early trials of heart failure, particularly the VHFT trials, upon which a great deal of our understanding of the pathogenesis of heart failure are based, in fact contained almost no women. The percentage of women in the SOLVD trial [75] that confirmed the benefit of ACE inhibitors varied from 11% in the prevention arm to 20% in the treatment arm. The highest percentage of women in an HF study was the 40% enrolled in the recent AHFT trial [60].

Much as we have presumed that all races would respond uniformly to all heart failure therapies, this concept has been shown to also be erroneous by gender. A retrospective review of over 7,000 patients enrolled in the international digoxin trial demonstrated that women had a worse outcome, with a 30% higher death from any cause in women (P = .014), a 28% higher

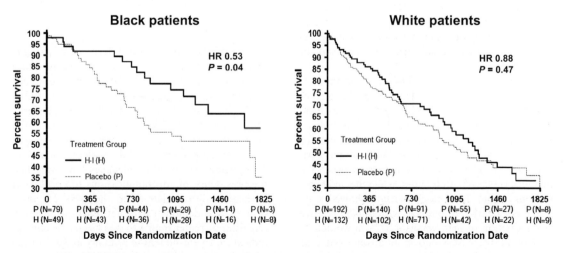

Fig. 5. Differing benefit of the combination of hydralazine and fixed dose nitrates on survival by race in the VHFT-1 trial. (*From* Carson P, Ziesche S, Johnson G, et al. Racial differences in response to therapy for heart failure: Analysis of the vasodilator-heart failure trials. J Card Fail 1999;5:178–87.)

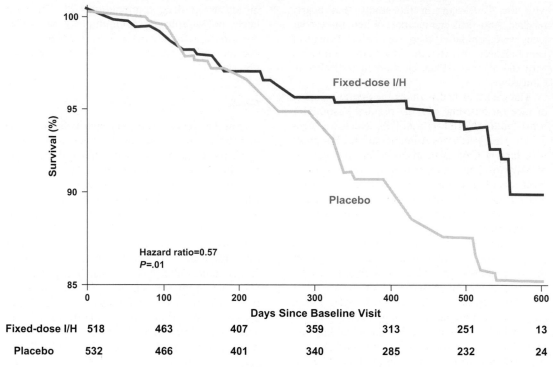

Fig. 6. Survival benefit on survival with the addition of hydralizine and fixed-dose nitrates over standard medical ther-apy in African Americans with heart failure in the AHFT trial. *Reproduced from* Taylor AL, Ziesche S, Yancy C, et al. Combination of Isosorbide dinitrate and hydralazine in blacks with heart failure. N Engl J Med 2004;351(20):2049–57; with permission.

incidence of cardiovascular death ($P = .035$), and a 38% higher likelihood of developing worsening heart failure ($P = .026$) when compared with men at the same age [79]. The hospitalizations because of heart failure were also 21% higher ($P = .01$) in women, demonstrating a higher over-all risk in women versus men who received di-goxin therapy.

Shelleke and colleagues [74] analyzed the out-come of various treatment trials for HF and com-pared the outcomes between women versus men. The results were not uniform. The study showed that there was a 10% relative worse outcome for women versus men in all of the ACE inhibitor tri-als (Fig. 7). The mean risk reduction was 18% in males versus 8% in females, while the difference in four recent beta-blocker trials showed only a 3% net relative difference, with a 34% relative risk reduction in men versus a 37% in women.

Not all drugs have shown an adverse outcome in women. Although there was an overall highly significant reduction in the relative risk of death with the hydralzine-nitrate therapy in the AHFT

trials compared with placebo, there was a signifi-cantly greater benefit in females than males (57% versus 39%) [80].

Comorbidities

One of the other major differences in patients enrolled in clinical trials, as opposed to those treated outside of clinical trials, is the prevalence of comorbidities, such as previous stroke, diabe-tes, hypertension, and particularly renal dysfunc-tion. Patients with these conditions are often excluded from the trials, whereas they represent a substantial percentage of the patients treated by a physician. Heiat and colleagues [55] examined the prevalence of contraindications to enrollment in heart failure trials over the past 15 years (Fig. 8), and demonstrated that renal insufficiency (creatinine greater than 1.6) was listed as a contra-indication to enrollment in as many as 30% of the trials between 1995 and 1999. Physicians and pharmaceutical companies interested in conduct-ing prospective trials evaluating a new drug or

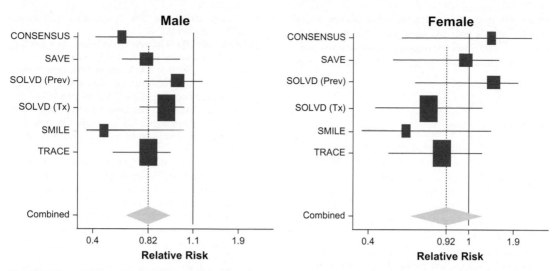

Fig. 7. Differing effect of ACE inhibitors by gender in clinical heart failure trials. *Abbreviations:* CONSENSUS, cooperative North Scandinavian enalapril survival study; SAVE, survival and ventricular enlargement; SMILE, survivors of myocardial infarction long-term evaluation; TRACE, trandolapril cardiac evaluation. *Reproduced from* Shekelle PG, Rich MW, Morton SC, et al. Efficacy of angiotensin-converting enzyme inhibitors and beta-blockers in the management of left ventricular systolic dysfunction according to race, gender, and diabetic status: a meta-analysis of major clinical trials. J Am College Cardiol 2003;41:1529–38; with permission.

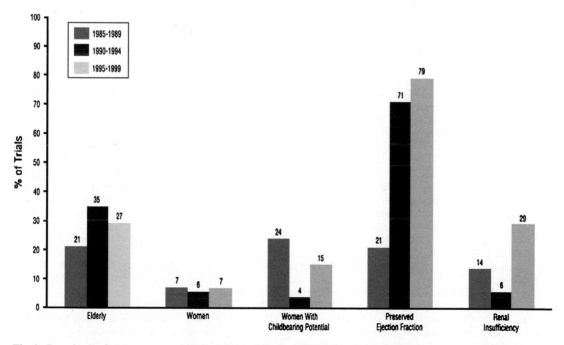

Fig. 8. Prevalence of common comorbidities in heart failure trials that have been contraindications to enrollment in clinical heart failure trials over time. From Heiat A, Gross CP, Krumholz HM. Representation of the elderly, women, and minorities in heart failure clinical trials. Arch Intern Med 2002;162;1682–8; with permission.

intervention are somewhat understandably reluctant to include patients with comorbidities, which may influence outcome and lead to erroneous conclusions about the potential benefit of that therapy.

Summary

There is a significant disparity between those treated and those studied with HF, including a significant lack of clinical trial data in some of the populations with the highest prevalence of the disease: females, African Americans, and Latinos, as well as those with preserved systolic function and those with common comorbidities. While retrospective reviews and sub group analysis may also be somewhat misleading, the results of many major trials upon which much of today's current therapy for HF are based may have shown different conclusions if balanced populations by race, gender, or potentially several comorbidities were included. Therefore, it seems that investigators cannot extrapolate all of the findings of clinical trials to patients in the general population. The important role of polymorphisms in gene expression and pharmacogenomics will also be important to a physician's approach to drug selection for individual patients in the future. Future trials of HF therapy will need to include a more representative sample from those more reflective of the expanding population with HF.

References

[1] American Heart Association Heart and Stoke Facts–2006 at AHA Heart Stoke Facts.

[2] Center for Disease Control and Health Statistics. Available at: http://CDC.org/Heartfailure/faststats/2006.

[3] Available at: http://UScensus.org.

[4] National Heart, Lung, and Blood Institute. Congestive heart failure data fact sheet. Available at: http://www.nhlbi.nih.gov/health/public/heart/other/CHF.htm. Accessed 2006.

[5] Redfield MM. Heart failure—an epidemic of uncertain proportions. N Engl J Med 2002;347(18):1442–4.

[6] Levy D, Kenchaiah S, Larson MG, et al. Long-term trends in the incidence of and survival with heart failure. N Engl J Med 2002;347(18):1397–402.

[7] Ammar KA, Jacobsen SJ, Mahoney DW, et al. Prevalence and prognostic significance of heart failure stages: application of the American College of Cardiology/American Heart Association heart failure staging criteria in the community. Circulation 2007;115(12):1563–70.

[8] Rodeheffer RJ. The new epidemiology of heart failure. Curr Cardiol Rep 2003;5(3):181–6.

[9] Roger VL, Weston SA, Redfield MM, et al. Trends in heart failure incidence and survival in a community-based population. JAMA 2004;292(3):344–50.

[10] Wang TJ, Evans JC, Benjamin EJ, et al. Natural history of asymptomatic left ventricular systolic dysfunction in the community. Circulation 2003;108(8):977–82.

[11] Senni M, Tribouilloy CM, Rodeheffer RJ, et al. Congestive heart failure in the community: trends in incidence and survival in a 10-year period. Arch Intern Med 1999;159(1):29–34.

[12] Goldberg RJ, Ciampa J, Lessard D, et al. Long-term survival after heart failure: a contemporary population-based perspective. Arch Intern Med 2007;167(5):490–6.

[13] Goldberg RJ, Spencer FA, Farmer C, et al. Incidence and hospital death rates associated with heart failure: a community-wide perspective. AM J Med 2005;118(7):728–34.

[14] Cowie MR, Wood DA, Coats AJ, et al. Survival of patients with a new diagnosis of heart failure: a population based study. Heart 2000;83(5):505–10.

[15] Jong P, Vowinckel E, Liu PP, et al. Prognosis and determinants of survival in patients newly hospitalized for heart failure: a population-based study. Arch intern Med 2006;220;162(15):1689–94.

[16] Shahar E, Lee S, Kim J, et al. Hospitalized heart failure: rates and long-term mortality. J Card Fail 2004;109(5):374–9.

[17] Cowie MR, Fox KF, Wood DA, et al. Hospitalization of patients with heart failure: a population-based study. Eur Heart J 2002;23(11):877–85.

[18] Pulignano G, Del Sindaco D, Tavazzi L, et al. for the IN-CHF Investigators. Clinical features and outcomes of elderly outpatients with heart failure followed up in hospital cardiology units: data from a large nationwide cardiology database (IN-CHF Registry). Am Heart J 2002;143(1):45–55.

[19] Fonarow GC, Gregg C, Heywood J, et al. ADHERE Scientific Advisory Committee and Investigators Temporal trends in clinical characteristics, treatments, and outcomes for heart failure hospitalizations, 2002 to 2004: findings from Acute Decompensated Heart Failure National Registry (ADHERE). Am Heart J 2007;153(6):1021–8.

[20] ADHERE. Insights from the ADHERE Registry Report 3.31.2006. Available at: http://www.adhereregistry.com. Accessed 2006.

[21] Adams KF, Sueta CA, Gheorghiade M, et al. Gender differences in survival in advanced heart failure: insights from the FIRST study. Circulation 1999;99:1816–21.

[22] Gold LD, Krumholz HM. Gender differences in treatment of heart failure and acute myocardial

infarction: a question of quality or epidemiology? Cardiol Rev 2006;14(4):180–6.

[23] Hoppe BL, Hermann DD. Sex differences in the causes and natural history of heart failure. Curr Cardiol Rep 2003;5(3):193–9.

[24] Yancy CW. Heart failure in African Americans. Am J Cardiol 2005;96(7B):3i–12i.

[25] Dries DL, Strong MH, Cooper RS, et al. Efficacy of angiotensin-converting enzyme inhibition in reducing progression from asymptomatic left ventricular dysfunction to symptomatic heart failure in black and white patients. J Am Coll Cardiol 2002;40(2): 311–7.

[26] Yancy CW. Heart failure therapy in special populations: the same or different? Rev Cardiovasc Med 2004;1(Suppl 5):S28–35.

[27] Owan TE, Hodge DO, Herges RM, et al. Trends in prevalence and outcome of heart failure with preserved ejection fraction. N Engl J Med 2006; 355(3):251–9.

[28] Bursi F, Weston SA, Redfield MM, et al. Systolic and diastolic heart failure in the community. JAMA 2006;296(18):2209–16.

[29] Vasan RS, Larson MG, Benjamin EJ, et al. Congestive heart failure in subjects with normal versus reduced left ventricular ejection fraction: prevalence and mortality in a population-based cohort. J Am Coll Cardiol 1999;33(7):1948–55.

[30] Yancy CW, Lopatin M, Stevenson LW, et al, for the ADHERE Scientific Advisory Committee and Investigators. Clinical presentation, management, and in-hospital outcomes of patients admitted with acute decompensated heart failure with preserved systolic function: a report from the Acute Decompensated Heart Failure National Registry (ADHERE) database. J Am Coll Cardiol 2006; 47(1):76–84.

[31] Owan TE, Redfield MM. Epidemiology of diastolic heart failure. Prog Cardiovasc Dis 2005;47(5): 320–32.

[32] Redfield MM, Jacobsen SJ, Burnett JC Jr, et al. Burden of systolic and diastolic ventricular dysfunction in the community: appreciating the scope of the heart failure epidemic. JAMA 2003;289(2): 194–202.

[33] Lenzen MJ, Scholte op Reimer WJ, Boersma E, et al. Differences between patients with a preserved and a depressed left ventricular function: a report from the Euro J Heart Failure 2004;25(14):1214–20.

[34] Thomas MD, Fox KF, Coats AJ, et al. The epidemiological enigma of heart failure with preserved systolic function. Eur J Heart Fail 2004;6(2):125–36.

[35] From AM, Leibson CL, Bursi F, et al. Diabetes in heart failure: prevalence and impact on outcome in the population. Am J Med 2006;119(7):591–9.

[36] Greenberg BH, Abraham WT, Albert NM, et al. Influence of diabetes on characteristics and outcomes in patients hospitalized with heart failure: a report from the Organized Program to Initiate Lifesaving Treatment in Hospitalized Patients with Heart Failure (OPTIMIZE-HF). Am Heart J 2007;154(2): 277e1–8.

[37] Fonarow GC, Horwich TB, Eshaghian S. Hemoglobin A1c and mortality: an unexpected relationship in patients with advanced heart failure. Am Heart J 2006;152(1):7–12.

[38] Smooke S, Horwich TB, Fonarow GC. Insulin-treated diabetes is associated with a marked increase in mortality in patients with advanced heart failure. Am Heart J 2005;149(1):168–74.

[39] Masoudi FA, Inzucchi SE. Diabetes mellitus and heart failure: epidemiology, mechanisms, and pharmacotherapy. Am J Cardiol 2007;99(4A):113B–32B.

[40] Artham SM, Lavie CJ, Milani RV, et al. The obesity paradox and discrepancy between peak oxygen consumption and heart failure prognosis—it's all in the fat. Congest Heart Fail 2007;13(3):177–80.

[41] Krumholz HM, Chen YT, Vaccarino V, et al. Correlates and impact on outcomes of worsening renal function in patients > 65 years of age with heart failure. Am J Cardiol 2000;85(9):1110–3.

[42] Patel J, Heywood JT. Management of the cardiorenal syndrome in heart failure. Curr Cardiol Rep 2006;8(3):211–6.

[43] Gottlieb SS, Abraham W, Butler J, et al. The prognostic importance of different definitions of worsening renal functions in congestive heart failure. J Card Fail 2002;8(3):136–41.

[44] Butler J, Forman DE, Abraham WT, et al. Relationship between heart failure treatment and development of worsening renal function among hospitalized patients. Am Heart J 2004;147(2): 331–8.

[45] Smith GL, Vaccarino V, Kosiborod M, et al. Worsening renal function: what is a clinically meaningful change in creatinine during hospitalization with heart failure? J Card Fail 2003;9(1):13–25.

[46] Smith GL, Shlipak MG, Havranek EP, et al. Serum urea nitrogen, creatinine, and estimators of renal function: mortality in older patients with cardiovascular disease. Arch Intern Med 2006;166(10): 1134–42.

[47] Fonarow GC, Adams KF Jr, Abraham WT, et al, ADHERE Scientific Advisory Committee, Study Group, and Investigators. Risk stratification for in-hospital mortality in acutely decompensated heart failure: classification and regression tree analysis. JAMA 2005;293(5):572–80.

[48] Levy WC, Mozaffarian D, Linker DT, et al. The Seattle heart failure model: prediction of survival in heart failure. Circulation 2006;113(11):1424–33.

[49] Cleland JG, Gennell I, Khound A, et al. Is the prognosis of heart failure improving? Eur J Heart Fail 1999;1(3):229–41.

[50] Hellermann JP, Goraya TY, Jacobsen SJ, et al. Incidence of heart failure after myocardial infarction: is it changing over time? Am J Epidemiol 2003;157(12): 1101–7.

[51] Stewart S, MacIntyre K, Hole DJ, et al. More "ma-lignant" than cancer? Five-year survival following a first admission for heart failure. Eur J Heart Fail 2001;3(3):315–22.

[52] National Cancer Institute. Cancer mortality maps & graphs Available at: http//www3.cancer. gov/atlasplus/charts.html. Accessed July 14, 2007.

[53] Poole-Wilson PA. Left ventricular dysfunction among elderly patients in general practice. Evidence based medicine is not yet possible in these patients. BMJ 1999;318(7196):1483–4.

[54] Gross CP, Mallory R, Heiat A, et al. Reporting the recruitment process in clinical trials: who are these patients and how did they get there? Ann Intern Med 2002;137(1):10–6.

[55] Heiat A, Gross CP, Krumholz HM. Representation of the elderly, women, and minorities in heart failure clinical trials. Arch Intern Med 2002;162:1682–8.

[56] Britton A, McKee M, Black N, et al. Threats to the applicability of randomized trails: exclusions and se-lective participation. J Health Serv Res Policy 1999; 4:112–21.

[57] Coca SG, Krumholz HM, Garg AX, et al. Under representation of renal disease in randomized con-trolled trials of cardiovascular disease. JAMA 2006;296(11):1377–84.

[58] Swedberg K, Cleland J, Dargie H, et al. Guidelines for the diagnosis and treatment of chronic heart fail-ure: executive summary (update 2005) European Society of Cardiology. Eur Heart J 2005;26(11): 1115–40.

[59] Hunt SA, Baker DW, Chin MH, et al, for the Amer-ican College of Cardiology/American Heart Associ-ation. ACC/AHA guidelines for the evaluation and management of chronic heart failure in the adult: ex-ecutive summary. J Am Coll Cardiol 2001;38(7): 2101–13.

[60] Taylor AL, Ziesche S, Yancy C, et al, African-Amer-ican Heart Failure Trial Investigators. Combination of isosorbide dinitrate and hydralazine in blacks with heart failure. N Engl J Med 2004;351(20):2049–57.

[61] Packer M, Fowler MB, Roecker EB, et al, for the Carvedilol Prospective Randomized Cumulative Sur-vival (COPERNICUS) Study Group. Effect of carve-dilol on the morbidity of patients with severe chronic heart failure. Circulation 2002;106(17):2194–9.

[62] Packer M, Bristow MR, Cohn JN. The effect of Car-vedilol on morbidity and mortality in patients with chronic heart failure. N Engl J Med 1996;334:1340–55.

[63] Pitt B. Evaluation of Losartan in the Elderly (ELITE) Trial: clinical implications. Eur Heart J 1997;18(8):1197–9.

[64] Yusuf S, Sleight P, Pogue J, et al. Effects of an angio-tensin-converting enzyme inhibitor, ramalpril, on cardiovascular events in high-risk patients. The Heart Outcomes Prevention Evaluation (HOPE) Study. N Engl J Med 2000;342:145–53.

[65] Young JB, Dunlap ME, Pfeffer MA, et al. Cande-sartan in Heart failure Assessment of Reduction in Mortality and Morbidity (CHARM) in patients with chronic heart failure and left ventricular sys-tolic dysfunction. Circulation 2004;110(17): 2618–26.

[66] The Beta-Blocker Evaluation of Survival Trial (BEST) Investigators. A trial of the beta-blocker Bucidilol in patients with advanced chronic heart failure. N Engl J Med 2001;344:1659–67.

[67] Konstam MA, Gheorghiade M, Burnett JC Jr. Effi-cacy of Vasopressin Antagonism in Heart Failure Outcome Study With Tolvaptan (EVEREST) in pa-tients hospitalized for worsening heart failure. JAMA 2007;297(12):1319–31.

[68] Celand JG, Daubert JC, Erdmann E. Cardiac Resynchronization-Heart Failure (CARE-HF) Study. The effect of cardiac resynchronization on morbidity and mortality in heart failure. N Engl J Med 2005;352(15):1539–49.

[69] Bardy GH, Lee KL, Mark DB. Sudden Cardiac death in Heart Failure Trail (SCD-HeFt) Amiodar-one or an implantable cardioverter-defibrillator for congestive heart failure. N Engl J Med 2005; 352(3):225–37.

[70] Rose EA, Gelijns AC, Moskowitz AJ, et al. Ran-domized Evaluation of Mechanical Assistance for the Treatment of Congestive Heart Failure (RE-MATCH) Study Group. N Engl J Med 2001; 345(20):1435–43.

[71] Rogers J, Kormos RL, Griffith BA, et al. Random-ized trial of pulsatile ventricular assist device versus medical therapy in patients who are inotrope depen-dent, the INTREPID Trial. J Am Coll Cardiol 2007; 50:741–7.

[72] Masoudi FA, Baillie CA, Wang Y. The complexity and cost of drug regimens of older patients hospital-ized with heart failure in the United States, 1998–2001. Arch Intern Med 2005;165(18):2069–76.

[73] Ko DT, Tu JV, Masoudi F. Quality of care and out-comes of older patients with heart failure hospital-ized in the United States and Canada. Arch Intern Med 2005;165(21):2486–92.

[74] Shekelle PG, Rich MW, Morton SC, et al. Efficacy of angiotensin-converting enzyme inhibitors and beta-blockers in the management of left ventricular systolic dysfunction according to race, gender, and diabetic status; a meta-analysis of major clinical trials. J Am Coll Cardiol 2003;41:1529–38.

[75] Effect of enalapril on survival in patients with re-duced left ventricular ejection fractions and conges-tive heart failure. The SOLVD investigators. N Engl J Med 1991;325:293–302.

[76] Exner DV, Dries DL, Domanski MJ, et al. Lesser re-sponse to angiotensin-converting enzyme inhibitor therapy in black as compared to white patients with left ventricular dysfunction. N Engl J Med 2001;344:1351–7.

[77] Cohn JN, Archibald DG, Ziesche S, et al. Effect of vasodilator therapy on mortality in chronic congres-tive heart failure: results of a Veterans

Administration Coorperative Study (V-HFT). N Engl J Med 1986;314:1547–52.

[78] Cohn JN, Loscalzo J, Franciosa JA. Nitric oxide's role in heart failure: pathophysiology and treatment. J Card Fail 2003;9(5):S197–8.

[79] Adams KF Jr, Patterson JH, Gattis WA, et al. Relationship of serum digoxin concentration to mortality and morbidity in women in the digitalis investigation group trial: a retrospective analysis. J Am Coll Cardiol 2005;46(3):497–504.

[80] Taylor AL, Lindenfeld J, Ziesche S, et al, A-HeFT Investigators. Outcomes by gender in the African-American heart failure trial. J Am Coll Cardiol 2006;48(11):2263–7.

Cardiol Clin 26 (2008) 127–135

Pharmacogenomics for Neurohormonal Intervention in Heart Failure

Dennis M. McNamara, MD*

University of Pittsburgh Medical Center, Pittsburgh, PA, USA

Variations useful to man...have undoubtedly occurred in the great and complex battle of life.
   Charles Darwin, *On the Origin of Species* [1].

After an initial myocardial injury, individuals progress to the syndrome of heart failure at markedly different rates, as noted by Sir William Osler over a century ago [2]. The myocardial injury elicits a complex systemic response involving the central nervous system, the kidney, and the vascular endothelium, collectively termed *neurohormonal activation*. The magnitude of this systemic response determines the rate of progression to the clinical syndrome. The advances of the human genome project have led to increased recognition of the inherent variation of important disease modifiers and the potential medical implications [3]. The clinical heterogeneity noted by Osler is to a great extent genetically based, because an individual's genetic background is a major determinant of the degree of neurohormonal activation.

Through modulating the neurohormonal response to injury, genetic background will influence heart failure progression and alter the impact of the pharmacologic therapy. Analysis of the critical genetic loci behind this "background effect" should facilitate individualized treatment decisions. To understand how pharmacogenetic interactions influence the impact of treatment, it is essential to begin with the main targets of current

pharmacotherapy: the angiotensin-converting enzyme (ACE) and the cardiac β-adrenergic receptors (βARs).

Angiotensin-converting enzyme deletion/insertion polymorphism

Heart failure outcomes

The ACE deletion/insertion (D/I) biallelic polymorphism of intron 16 is the most extensively studied cardiovascular polymorphism, and has been the subject of hundreds of investigations since its initial discovery [4,5]. Although the clinical implications of this polymorphism have been controversial, the physiologic association of the ACE D/I polymorphism with enzymatic activity has been consistent. The D allele has been linked in nearly every clinical study to increased activity of ACE and higher levels of the product of ACE activity, the peptide mediator angiotensin II (a2) [6]. The cellular mechanism is unknown, but this linkage of genotype with ACE activity is consistent across different clinical paradigms from hypertension to myocardial infarction [7–9] and demonstrates a D allele "dose effect" for a2 levels. Subjects with the DD genotype have the highest levels of a2, heterozygotes are intermediate, and those homozygous for I allele have the lowest levels. For disease states such as heart failure, where a2 facilitates disease progression, the potential implications of this genetically "ordered" ACE activity are apparent.

Given the role of renin-angiotensin activation in heart failure, it is hypothesized that the ACE D allele functions as a genetic modifier, accelerates disease progression, and worsens survival. This has been demonstrated in three clinical

A version of this article originally appeared in Heart Failure Clinics, volume 1, issue 1.

This article was supported in part by National Institute of Health Grants HL 69912 and HL 075038.

* Heart Failure/Transplantation Program, University of Pittsburgh Medical Center, S-558 Lothrop Street, Pittsburgh, PA 15213

E-mail address: mcnamaradm@upmc.edu

investigations. The first, a study of 193 subjects who had idiopathic dilated cardiomyopathy, demonstrated poorer survival for subjects homozygous for the D allele [10]. Most recently, the adverse impact of the ACE D allele was demonstrated in 978 subjects post–myocardial infarction [11]. The impact in this cohort was primarily in subjects who had lower left ventricular ejections fraction (LVEF) or higher brain naturetic peptide levels. Forty-five percent of the subjects in the post–myocardial infarction study were on ACE inhibitor therapy, compared with only 25% of subjects in the study of idiopathic dilated cardiomyopathy. Neither study addressed the potential pharmacogenetic interactions of the ACE D/I polymorphism with the medical therapy of heart failure.

Pharmacogenetics of the angiotensin-converting enzyme deletion/insertion polymorphism: Genetic Risk Assessment of Cardiac Events

A similar overall impact of the ACE D allele on heart failure outcomes was demonstrated in a study at the University of Pittsburgh, the GRACE study of Genetic Risk Assessment of Cardiac Events. Four hundred seventy-nine subjects who had systolic dysfunction (mean LVEF 0.25 ± 0.08) with ischemic and nonischemic etiologies were followed for a median of 3 years until death or cardiac transplantation. The D allele was associated with poorer transplant-free survival, and demonstrated the same "gene-ordered" effect shown for ACE activity: II homozygotes demonstrated the best survival, DD homozygotes the poorest, and heterozygotes showed the predicted "intermediate" survival between the homozygotes. The adverse impact of the D allele on survival for this cohort first was reported on an analysis of the first 328 subjects [12], and remained evident during analysis of the entire cohort (Fig. 1) [13].

β-*Blocker therapy*

Genetic background must interact with environment, and for the heart failure patient a critical aspect of the local "environment" is the pharmacologic milieu. GRACE examined how pharmacologic inhibition may alter the effect of genetic modulation of neurohormonal activation on heart failure outcomes. Ninety-five percent of subjects in GRACE were on ACE inhibitors or a2 receptor blockers (ARBs), whereas only 42% were on β-blockers, reflecting the evolution of care when

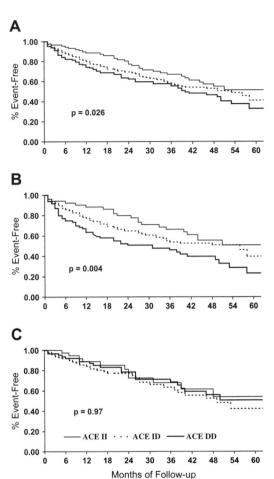

Fig. 1. Transplant-free survival by ACE D/I genotype, GRACE study, University of Pittsburgh. (*A*) Overall cohort, ACE D allele associated with poorer event-free survival (n = 479, *P* = .026). (*B*) Subset with no β-blocker therapy (n = 277, *P* = .004). (*C*) Subset treated with β-blocker therapy (n = 202, *P* = .97). (*From* McNamara DM, Holubkov R, Postava L, et al. Phamacogenetic interactions between ACE inhibitor therapy and the angiotensin-converting enzyme deletion polymorphism in patients with congestive heart failure. J Amer Coll Cardiol 2004;44:2019–26; with permission.)

the study began. For β-blockers, analysis by treatment subset demonstrated the effects of ACE D on outcomes to be primarily in subjects not treated with β-blockers [12,13] and that β-blocker therapy eliminates the impact of the polymorphism (see Fig. 1). For subjects not on β-blockers, the 2-year event-free survival for DD subjects was 51%, versus 80% for the II homozygotes. In contrast, for subjects on β-blockers, no effect of the D allele on outcomes was apparent.

The elimination of the effect of the D allele by β-blocker therapy likely reflects their role as inhibitors of renin release. Sympathetic activation is an important stimulus to the renin angiotensin activity in heart failure, and β-blockers markedly reduce a2 levels [14].

The potential usefulness of this pharmacogenetic interaction is evident when examining the impact of β-blocker therapy within ACE D/I genetic subsets (Fig. 2). Although β-blockers improved survival overall in the GRACE cohort, much of that benefit is in the DD homozygotes genetically predicted to have the highest levels of ACE activity. The impact of therapy is diminished in the heterozygotes, and in this small cohort is no longer evident for subjects who are II homozygotes. These results suggest the ACE D/I polymorphism delineates genetic subsets of heart failure patients in whom the therapeutic impact of β-blockade on heart failure survival is different. A recent study [15] of the effect of β-blockers in 199 subjects who had chronic heart failure demonstrated similar improvements in LVEF in all three genetic subsets, and suggests the ACE D/I polymorphism does not predict this particular endpoint of β-blocker response.

Angiotensin-converting enzyme inhibitor therapy

Based on ACE activity, it is predicted that the ACE D/I polymorphisms should modulate the effect of ACE inhibitors. Because 95% of the subjects in GRACE were on either an ACE inhibitor or an ARB, this pharmacogenetic interaction was investigated in this cohort using a dose analysis comparing the effect of higher dose ACE therapy (>50% of target daily dose defined by national guidelines) on transplant-free survival to low-dose therapy (≤50%). This resulted in a roughly threefold difference in the mean dose for the high-dose group compared with the low-dose group. In contrast, the multicenter Assessment of Treatment with Lisinopril and Survival (ATLAS) trial [16] evaluated the impact of a 10-fold difference in the mean dose of ACE inhibitor. Analysis by ACE dose treatment subset suggests higher doses of ACE inhibitors limit the adverse impact of the ACE D allele [13], and this effect of high-dose therapy was particularly evident in subjects not treated with β-blockers (Fig. 3).

In overall event-free survival, the benefits of higher dose ACE inhibitors were modest with the

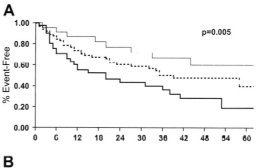

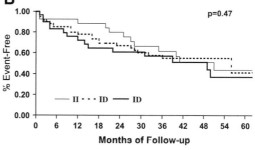

Fig. 3. Transplant-free survival by ACE D/I genotype, GRACE study, University of Pittsburgh. (*A*) Subset on low-dose ACE inhibitors and no β-blockers. ACE D allele was associated with poorer event-free survival (n = 130, P = .005). (*B*) Subset with high-dose ACE inhibitor therapy and no β-blockers (n = 117, P = .47). (*Data from* McNamara DM, Holubkov R, Postava L, et al. Phamacogenetic interactions between ACE inhibitor therapy and the angiotensin-converting enzyme deletion polymorphism in patients with congestive heart failure. J Amer Coll Cardiol 2004;44:2019–26; with permission.)

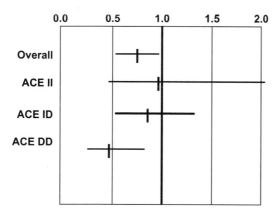

Fig. 2. Relative risk of event (death or transplantation) by β-blocker use, GRACE study: overall cohort and by ACE D/I, DD, DI, and II genotype. (*Data from* McNamara DM, Holubkov R, Postava L, et al. Phamacogenetic interactions between ACE inhibitor therapy and the angiotensin-converting enzyme deletion polymorphism in patients with congestive heart failure. J Amer Coll Cardiol 2004;44:2019–26.)

relative risk (RR) of high-dose therapy 0.88. This 12% reduction was not statistically significant, but was similar to the trend in survival benefit seen in ATLAS. The RR reduction with higher dose ACE inhibitor therapy within ACE genotype class demonstrated a gene-ordered effect similar to that seen with β-blockers, with the greatest impact within the DD subset, although this failed to reach significance (Fig. 4).

The effect of high-dose therapy in DD homozygotes is consistent with greater resistance to ACE inhibition in this subset. In subjects who have heart failure, the blood pressure response to captopril demonstrates minimal effects in DD subjects, an intermediate response in heterozygotes, and the greatest impact in II patients [17]. A similar interaction was demonstrated for chronic therapy with angiotensin-receptor antagonists in hypertensive subjects [18]. The studies suggest a diminished response to ACE inhibition or blockade with the ACE D allele. The higher ACE activity evident in ACE DD homozygotes is the most likely mechanism of this genetically determined drug "resistance."

Aldosterone receptor antagonists

The prevalence of "aldosterone escape" on ACE inhibitors is greatest in the ACE DD genotype [19]. The impact of the aldosterone receptor antagonist spironolactone on left ventricular remodeling also is diminished in the ACE DD subset compared with the ID and II subsets [20],

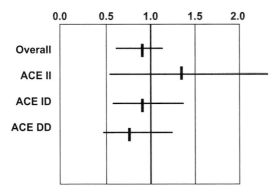

Fig. 4. Relative risk of event (death or transplantation) by ACE inhibitor dose use, GRACE study: overall cohort and by ACE D/I, DD, DI, and II genotype. (*Adapted from* McNamara DM, Holubkov R, Postava L, et al. Phamacogenetic interactions between ACE inhibitor therapy and the angiotensin-converting enzyme deletion polymorphism in patients with congestive heart failure. J Amer Coll Cardiol 2004;44:2019–26; with permission.)

closely paralleling the diminished clinical response to ACE inhibitors. The influence of the ACE D/I polymorphism on the effect of aldosterone receptor antagonists on survival remains to be determined.

β-Adrenergic receptor variation

Although the ACE D/I polymorphism is an important component, neurohormonal activation is polygenic and variation at multiple loci will determine the overall impact of genetic background on heart failure treatment. Genetic variation in the cellular targets of pharmacologic therapy predicts several genomic loci as potential major determinants of this "background effect." The impact of β-blockers is mediated through β_1- and β_2-adrenergic receptors, and the functional significance of their common genetic polymorphisms has been researched intensely [21].

Structure and function

Activation of both β receptor subtypes is linked to increased cyclic adenosine monophosphate (cAMP) formation through the interaction with stimulatory guanine nucleotide-binding protein (G_s). In the normal heart, β_1 receptors predominate over β_2 receptors at a ratio of approximately 4:1, whereas in the failing myocardium, sympathetic overactivation leads to selective downregulation of β_1 receptors to a greater extent than β_2; as a result, the percentage of β_2 receptors may increase up to 40% [22]. In contrast, β_2 receptors do not decrease in receptor number, but become deactivated or less responsive to agonist stimulation.

The β_1-adrenergic receptor (Fig. 5) is encoded for by an intronless gene and consists of a protein with 477 amino acid residues and seven transmembrane domains (TMDs). The first 60 amino acids of the amino terminus comprise the extracellular surface of the receptor, whereas the final 90 amino acids are located in the cytoplasmic domain. The β_2 receptor subtype (Fig. 6) has a similar genomic and protein structure [23] with a coding region of 1239 nucleic acids encoding for 413 amino acids. Between β_1 and β_2 adrenergic receptors, the greatest amino acid identity (71%) is found in the TMDs, and the tertiary structure in the lipid bilayer takes on a ring or barrel shape that allows for multiple ligand contact points [24]. The cytoplasmic regions of the two receptor classes are more distinct, which allows for more

Beta₁ Adrenergic Receptor

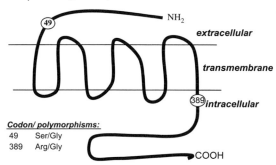

Codon/ polymorphisms:
49   Ser/Gly
389   Arg/Gly

Fig. 5. Structure of the β₁ adrenergic receptor: common polymorphisms. Arg, arginine; COOH, carboxyl terminus; Gly, glycine; NH2, amino terminus; Ser, serine. (*From* McNamara DM, MacGowan GA, London B. Clinical importance of beta adrenoceptor polymorphisms in cardiovascular disease. Am J Pharmacogenomics 2002;2: 73–8; with permission.)

diversity in their signaling interactions with other intracellular proteins [25].

Functional variation and heart failure outcomes: β₂

Initial investigations of functional genetic variation focused on the β₂ receptor because of its importance in the pharmacologic treatment of asthma [26]. Population studies have revealed three common polymorphisms resulting in an amino acid substitution–Arg16Gly, Glu27Gln, and Thr164Ile–and in vitro studies have

Beta₂ Adrenergic Receptor

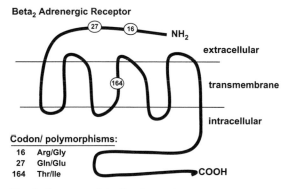

Codon/ polymorphisms:
16   Arg/Gly
27   Gln/Glu
164   Thr/Ile

Fig. 6. Structure of the β₂ adrenergic receptor: common polymorphisms. Arg, arginine; COOH, carboxyl terminus; Gln, glutamine; Glu, glutamate; Gly, glycine; Ile, Isoleucine; NH2, amino terminus; Thr, threonine. (*From* McNamara DM, MacGowan GA, London B. Clinical importance of beta adrenoceptor polymorphisms in cardiovascular disease. Am J Pharmacogenomics 2002;2: 73–8; with permission.)

demonstrated significant functional consequences in terms of receptor function or regulation [27]. The substitution of Ile for Thr occurs with allele frequency of approximately 3% to 5%, and the Ile164 receptor has significantly lower binding affinity for isoproterenol, epinephrine, and norepinephrine (Table 1) [28]. Agonist stimulation of the Ile variant produces a lower level of adenylyl cyclase activity with the Thr wild type receptor. Examination of murine models seems consistent with in vitro studies, because transgenic mice that overexpress the Ile164 receptor in the heart have a decrease in resting and (agonist-stimulated) contractile function in vivo compared with transgenic controls overexpressing the wild type Thr164 receptor [29].

The functional significance of the Ile164 variant in vitro and in animal models supports a potential clinically significant role in heart failure, which has been demonstrated in clinical outcomes studies. A prospective study at the University of Cincinnati of 259 patients who had class II–IV heart failure found that the presence of the Ile164 receptor polymorphism markedly decreased transplant-free survival with an RR for death or transplant of 4.8 compared with those homozygous for Thr164 [30]. Investigation in this population also revealed a marked reduction in functional capacity, as measured by metabolic stress testing, among patients with the Ile 164 [31]. A study of normal Thr164Ile heterozygotes demonstrated blunted agonist responsiveness compared with subjects homozygous for Thr164 [32,33], which may underlie its adverse impact on heart failure survival.

The effect of the Ile164 variant in these investigations supports the importance of the β₂ receptor in heart failure progression, although the small number of subjects with the variant limits pharmacogenetic investigations. Several studies have linked the more common Arg16Gly or Glu27Gln polymorphisms to hypertension [34,35], but no influence on heart failure outcomes has been shown [30].

Functional variation and heart failure outcomes: β₁

The two most common polymorphisms for the β₁ receptor are Ser49Gly and Arg389Gl [36], and both seem to be linked to heart failure outcomes. The relative allele frequency for the Arg389Gly variant is approximately 0.70/0.30, and for the Ser49Gly polymorphism 0.85/0.15.

Table 1
Frequency and function of β_1 and β_2 polymorphisms

Codon	Region	Polymorphism	Allele frequency (%)	Function in vitro
β_1				
389	Cytoplasmic	Arg/Gly	70/30	Arg: gain of function (increased cAMP)
49	Extracellular	Ser/Gly	85/15	No data
β_2				
16	Extracellular	Arg/Gly	40/60	Gly: enhanced downregulation
27	Extracellular	Gln/Glu	55/45	Glu: resistance to downregulation
164	Transmembrane domain 4	Thr/Ile	95/5	Ile: loss of function, decreased agonist binding, decreased cAMP

Abbreviations: Arg, arginine; Gln, glutamine; Glu, glutamate; Gly, glycine; Ile, isoleucine; Ser, serine; Thr, threonin.
Adapted from McNamara DM, MacGowan GA, London B. Clinical importance of beta adrenoceptor polymorphisms in cardiovascular disease. Am J Pharmacogenomics 2002;2:73–8; with permission.

The codon 49 polymorphism is located in the extracellular domain of the receptor (see Fig. 5), and the Gly49 variant is associated in vitro with increased receptor down-regulation [37,38]. In contrast, amino acid 389 is located near the carboxyl-terminus cytoplasmic tail and in vitro demonstrates a higher basal adenylyl cyclase activity with the Arg389 receptor. With agonist stimulation this distinction was magnified greatly, suggesting the Arg389 variant results in a gain of function for G-protein coupling [39].

An examination of more than 1000 normal individuals suggested that the Gly49 variant was associated with lower resting heart rate [40]. A heart failure outcomes study in 184 subjects who had systolic dysfunction suggested the Gly49 variant was associated with improved survival [41]. An examination of the GRACE cohort suggests the Gly49 variant is linked to greater benefit from adrenergic receptor blockade [42]. The Arg389 variant was linked to a greater risk for heart failure in an African-American cohort, but only when co-inherited with a deletion of the α-2C receptor [43]. The genetic substudy of the BEST trial of bucindilol suggests the presence of the 389Arg variant predicts a greater improvement of survival with β-blocker therapy [44], but this linkage of 389Arg to β-blocker benefit was not evident with metoprolol in the MERIT-HF substudy [45]. In a similar fashion, examination of the impact of 389Arg on blood pressure response in hypertensive subjects has led to conflicting results [46,47].

Endothelial nitric oxide synthase

Nitric oxide (NO) plays an important protective role in heart failure [48,49] and endothelial nitric oxide synthase (NOS3) is the predominant source of vascular NO. A common polymorphism (G894T) exists on exon 7 (codon 298: Glu298Asp) for which the wild type glutamate is replaced with aspartic acid [50]. The functional role of this apparently charge-neutral amino acid change is controversial, but the Asp298 variant has a shorter half-life and therefore less NO activity in endothelial cell culture [51]. The Asp298 variant has been linked to the risk for coronary disease, hypertension, and stroke. For subjects who had heart failure, functional assessment by metabolic stress testing demonstrated significantly higher maximum oxygen consumption in subjects who had the Glu298Glu phenotype compared with those homozygous or heterozygous for the Asp298 variant [52]. This modulation of functional capacity by the Asp298Glu polymorphism parallels the impact on survival, because poorer transplant-free survival was evident for subjects with the Asp298 variant compared with individuals homozygous for Glu298 (Fig. 7) [52]. Although the Asp298 variant has been investigated as a risk factor for coronary disease, the impact in GRACE reflects a role as a modulator of heart failure, and was more apparent in the nonischemic cohort.

Pharmacogenetic interactions with endothelial nitric oxide synthase and angiotensin-converting enzyme inhibitors

Clinical and animal studies demonstrate that NOS3 plays a central role in the therapeutic effects of ACE inhibitors. Murine knockout models have demonstrated that the postinfarction benefit of ACE inhibitors on remodeling depends on NOS3 [53]. In clinical studies of vascular reactivity, the effects of ACE inhibitors are diminished

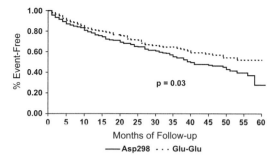

Fig. 7. Transplant-free survival by NOS3 codon 298 polymorphism, GRACE study, University of Pittsburgh. Overall cohort (n = 469): Asp[298] variant (*solid line*), n = 266; Glu[298] homozygotes (*dashed line*), n = 203. Event-free survival was significantly poorer in subjects with the Asp[298] variant ($P = .03$). (*From* McNamara DM, Holubkov R, Postava L, et al. The Asp[298] variant of endothelial nitric oxide synthase: effect on survival for patients with congestive heart failure. Circulation 2003;107:1598–602; with permission.)

by pretreatment with NOS inhibitors. In GRACE, the examination of high-dose versus low-dose ACE inhibitor suggests a pharmacogenetic interaction with the NOS3 Glu298Asp polymorphism, because the impact of Asp298 was primarily in subjects on low-dose ACE inhibitor, and was not evident in those receiving high-dose therapy [54]. Analysis of the impact of ACE inhibitor dose by genetic subset suggests the variable benefit of ACE inhibitors may be explained partially by variation at the NOS3 locus, but this will need additional investigation in larger cohorts.

Summary

For the ACE D/I polymorphism, linkage of the D allele to higher ACE activity results in a predictable impact for therapies inhibiting a2 production: ACE inhibitors and β-receptor antagonists. Both therapies seem to have their greatest impact on the 30% of the population who are homozygous for the D allele, genetically predicted to have the highest levels of neurohormonal activation. Several independent groups of investigators have demonstrated the adverse impact of the ACE D allele in heart failure, which is consistent with the role of renin-angiotensin activation in clinical progression. Genotyping of the ACE locus may identify large subsets of patients who receive maximal benefit for aggressive neurohormonal blockade.

Predictably, genetic influences on heart failure therapy are polygenic. In addition to ACE, the therapeutic impact of β-receptor antagonists is influenced by variation at the β_1 receptor locus. The effectiveness of ACE inhibitor therapy may be influenced by variation of ACE and NOS3. Pharmacogenetic investigations have not integrated more than one genetic loci into a clinical outcomes model, and larger cohorts will be required for adequate statistical power to address polygenic "background" effects. Analysis of genetic background has become a potential clinical tool for predicting heart failure outcomes and targeting therapeutic intervention. Prospective validation of the predictive impact of genetic variants will be required before the routine implementation of genetically individualized treatments.

References

[1] Darwin C. Natural selection. In: On the origin of species. London: J. Murray; 1859. p. 80.
[2] Osler W. Diseases of the circulatory system. In: The principles and practice of medicine. New York: D. Appleton and Co.; 1892. p. 623–40.
[3] Ligget SB. Pharmacogenetic applications of the human genome project. Nat Med 2001;7:281–3.
[4] Rigat B, Hubert C, Alhenc-Gelas F, et al. An insertion/deletion polymorphism in the angiotensin I-converting enzyme gene accounting for half the variance of serum enzyme levels. J Clin Invest 1990;86:1343–6.
[5] Rigat B, Hubert C, Corvol P, et al. PCR detection of the insertion/deletion polymorphism of the human angiotensin converting enzyme gene (DCP) (dipeptidyl carboxypeptidase 1). Nucleic Acids Res 1992; 20:1433.
[6] Tiret L, Rigat B, Visvikis S, et al. Evidence, from combined segregation and linkage analysis, that a variant of the angiotensin I-converting enzyme (ACE) gene controls plasma ACE levels. Am J Hum Genet 1992;51:197–205.
[7] Danser AH, Derkx FH, Hense HW, et al. Angiotensinogen (M235T) and angiotensin-converting enzyme (I/D) polymorphisms in association with plasma renin and prorenin levels. J Hypertens 1998;16:1879–83.
[8] Cambien F, Poirier O, Lecerf L, et al. Deletion polymorphism in the gene for angiotensin-converting enzyme is a potent risk factor for myocardial infarction. Nature 1992;359:641–4.
[9] Ihnken R, Verho K, Gross M, et al. Deletion polymorphism of the angiotensin I-converting enzyme gene is associated with increased plasma angiotensin-converting enzyme activity but not with increased risk for myocardial infarction and

coronary artery disease. Ann Intern Med 1996; 125(1):19–25.

[10] Andersson B, Sylven C. The DD genotype of the angiotensin-converting enzyme gene is associated with increased mortality in idiopathic heart failure. J Am Coll Cardiol 1996;28:162–7.

[11] Palmer BR, Pilbrow AP, Yandle TG, et al. Angiotensin-converting enzyme gene polymorphism interacts with left ventricular ejection fraction and brain natriuretic peptide levels to predict mortality after myocardial infarction. J Am Coll Cardiol 2003;41: 729–36.

[12] McNamara DM, Holubkov R, Janosko K, et al. Pharmacogenetic interactions between β-blocker therapy and the angiotensin-converting enzyme deletion polymorphism in patients with congestive heart failure. Circulation 2001;103:1644–8.

[13] McNamara DM, Holubkov R, Postava L, et al. Phamacogenetic interactions between ACE inhibitor therapy and the angiotensin-converting enzyme deletion polymorphism in patients with congestive heart failure. J Amer Coll Cardiol 2004;44:2019–26.

[14] Campbell D, Aggrarwal A, Esler M, et al. Beta blockers, angiotenisn II, and ACE inhibitors in patients with heart failure. Lancet 2001;358:1609–10.

[15] de Groote P, Helbecque N, Lamblin N, et al. Beta-adrenergic receptor blockade and the angiotensin-converting enzyme deletion polymorphism in patients with chronic heart failure. Eur J Heart Fail 2004;6:17–21.

[16] Packer M, Poole-Wilson PA, Armstrong PW, et al. Comparative effects of low and high doses of the angiotensin-converting enzyme inhibitor, lisinopril, on morbidity and mortality in chronic heart failure. Circulation 1999;100:2312–8.

[17] O'Toole L, Stewart M, Padfield P, et al. Effect of the insertion/deletion polymorphism of the angiotensin-converting enzyme gene on the response to angiotensin-converting inhibitors in patients with heart failure. J Cardiovasc Pharmacol 1998;32:988–94.

[18] Kurland L, Melhus H, Karlsson J, et al. Angiotensin-converting enzyme gene polymorphism predicts blood pressure response to angiotensin II receptor type 1 antagonist treatment in hypertensive patients. J Hypertens 2001;19:1783–7.

[19] Cicoira M, Zanolla L, Rossi A, et al. Failure of aldosterone suppression despite angiotensin-converting enzyme (ACE) inhibitor administration in chronic heart failure associated with the ACE DD genotype. J Am Coll Cardiol 2001;37:1808–12.

[20] Ciocoira M, Rossi A, Bonapace S, et al. Effects of ACE gene insertion/deletion polymorphism on response to sprironolactone in patients with chronic heart failure. Am J Med 2004;116:657–61.

[21] McNamara DM, MacGowan GA, London B. Clinical importance of beta adrenoceptor polymorphisms in cardiovascular disease. Am J Pharmacogenomics 2002;2:73–8.

[22] Bristow MR. Beta adrenergic receptor blockade in the failing heart. Circulation 2000;101:558–69.

[23] Buscher R, Herrmann V, Insel PA. Human adrenoceptor polymorphisms: evolving recognition of clinical importance. Trends Pharmacol Sci 1999;20: 94–9.

[24] Steinberg SF. The molecular basis for distinct beta adrenergic receptor subtype action in cardiomyocytes. Circ Res 1999;85:1101–11.

[25] Lefkowitz RF, Rockman HA, Koch WJ. Catecholamines, cardiac beta adrenergic receptors and heart failure. Circulation 2000;101:1634–7.

[26] Liggett SB. Pharmacogenetics of relevant targets in asthma. Clin Exp Allergy 1998;28:77–9.

[27] Liggett SB. β2 adrenergic receptor pharmacogenetics. Am J Respir Crit Care Med 2000;161: S197–201.

[28] Green SA, Cole G, Jacinto M, et al. A polymorphism of the beta 2-adrenergic receptor within the fourth membrane domain alters ligand binding and functional properties of the receptor. J Biol Chem 1993;268:23116–21.

[29] Turki J, Lorenz JN, Green SA, et al. Myocardial signaling defects and impaired cardiac function of human beta 2-adrenergic receptor polymorphism expressed in transgenic mice. Proc Natl Acad Sci USA 1996;93:10483–8.

[30] Liggett SB, Wagoner LE, Craft LL, et al. The Ile164 β2 adrenergic receptor polymorphism adversely affects the outcome of congestive heart failure. J Clin Invest 1998;102:1534–9.

[31] Wagoner LE, Craft LL, Singh B, et al. Polymorphisms of the β2 adrenergic receptor determine exercise capacity in patients with heart failure. Circ Res 2000;86:834–40.

[32] Brodde OE, Busher R, Tellkamp R, et al. Blunted cardiac responses to receptor activation in subjects with Thr164Ile β2 adrenoceptors. Circulation 2001; 103:1048–50.

[33] Feldman RD. Adrenergic receptor polymorphisms in cardiac function (and dysfunction): a failure to communicate? Circulation 2001;1003:1042–3.

[34] Timmermann B, Mo R, Lutt FC, et al. β2 adrenoceptor genetic variation is associated with genetic predisposition to essential hypertension: the Bergen blood pressure study. Kidney Int 1998;53:1455–60.

[35] Busjahn A, Li GH, Faulhaber HD, et al. β2 adrenergic receptor gene variations, blood pressure, and heart size in normal twins. Hypertension 2000;35: 555–62.

[36] Maqbool A, Hall AS, Paul SG, et al. Common polymorphisms of β1 adrenoceptor: identification and rapid screening assay. Lancet 1999;353:897–9.

[37] Levin MC, Marullo S, Muntaner O, et al. The myocardium protective variant of the Gly-49 variant of the beta 1 adrenergic receptor exhibits constitutive activity and increased desensitization and downregulation. J Biol Chem 2002;34:30429–35.

[38] Rathz DA, Brown KM, Kramer LA, et al. Amino acid 49 polymorphisms of the human beta 1 adrenergic receptor affect agonist promoted trafficking. J Cardiovasc Pharmacol 2002;39:155–260.

[39] Mason DA, Moore JD, Green SA, et al. A gain of function polymorphism in a g-protein coupling domain of the human β_1 adrenergic receptor. J Biol Chem 1999;274:12670–4.

[40] Ranade K, Jorgenson E, Sheu WH, et al. A polymorphism in the beta 1 receptor is associated with resting heart rate. Am J Hum Genet 2002;70: 935–42.

[41] Borjesson M, Magnusson Y, Hjalmarson A, et al. A novel polymorphism in the gene coding for the β_1 adrenergic receptor associated with survival in patients with heart failure. Eur Heart J 2000;21: 1810–2.

[42] Postava L, Mahlab D, Holubkov R, et al. β1 and β2 Adrenergic receptor polymorphisms and heart failure survival: interaction with beta blockade [abstract]. Circulation 2002;19(Suppl):II–611.

[43] Liggett SB, Wagoner LE, Levin AM, et al. Synergistic polymorphisms of beta 1 and alpha 2c adrenergic receptors and the risk of congestive heart failure. N Engl J Med 2002;347:1135–42.

[44] Liggett S.B. Late Breaking Clinical Trials. Presented at the Heart Failure Society of America. Toronto, September, 2004.

[45] White HL, de Boar RA, Maqbool A, et al. An evaluation of the beta-1 adrenergic receptor Arg389Gly polymorphism in individuals with heart failure: a MERIT-HF sub-study. Eur J Heart Fail 2003;5: 463–8.

[46] Johnson JA, Zineh I, Puckett BJ, et al. Beta-1 adrenergic receptor polymorphisms and antihypertensive response to metoprolol. Clin Pharmacol Ther 2003; 74:44–52.

[47] Brodde OR, Stein CM. The Gly389Arg beta 1 adrenergic receptor polymorphism: a predictor of response to beta-blocker treatment? Clin Pharmacol Ther 2003;74:299–302.

[48] Kelly RA, Balligand JL, Smith TW. Nitric oxide and cardiac function. Circ Res 1996;79:363–80.

[49] Drexler H. Nitric oxide synthases in the failing human heart: a double-edged sword? Circulation 1999;99:2972–5.

[50] Philip I, Plantefeve G, Vuillaumier-Barrot S, et al. G894T polymorphism in the endothelial nitric oxide synthase gene is associated with an enhanced vascular responsiveness to phenylephrine. Circulation 1999;99:3096–8.

[51] Tesauro M, Thompson WC, Rogliani P, et al. Intracellular processing of endothelial nitric oxide synthase isoforms associated with differences in severity of cardiopulmonary diseases: cleavage of proteins with aspartate vs. glutamate at position 298. Proc Natl Acad Sci USA 2000;97:2832–5.

[52] McNamara DM, Holubkov R, Postava L, et al. The Asp[298] variant of endothelial nitric oxide synthase: effect on survival for patients with congestive heart failure. Circulation 2003;107:1598–602.

[53] Yang XP, Liu YH, Sheseley EG, et al. Endothelial nitric oxide gene knockout mice cardiac phenotypes and the effect of angiotensin-converting enzyme inhibitor on myocardial ischemia/reperfusion injury. Hypertension 1999;34:24–30.

[54] Bedi M, Murali S, MacGowan G, et al. High dose ACE inhibitors reduces the impact of the NOS3 Asp298 variant on heart failure survival. Circulation 2003;1085 IV–444.

Index

Note: Page numbers of article titles are in **boldface** type.